GENTLE EATING

EATING

WORKBOOK

GENTLE EATING
WORKBOOK

STEPHEN ARTERBURN, M.ED.,
AND VIVIAN LAMPHEAR, PH.D.
WITH SHERRY MARLAR

OLIVER
NELSON

THOMAS NELSON PUBLISHERS
Nashville • Atlanta • London • Vancouver

Published in Nashville, Tennessee, by Thomas Nelson, Inc., Publishers, and distributed in Canada by Word Communications, Ltd., Richmond, British Columbia.

Unless otherwise noted, the Bible version used in this publication is THE NEW KING JAMES VERSION. Copyright © 1979, 1980, 1982, Thomas Nelson, Inc., Publishers. Verses marked TLB are taken from *The Living Bible,* copyright 1971 by Tyndale House Publishers, Wheaton, IL. Used by permission.

ISBN 0-7852-7520-7

Printed in the United States of America
1 2 3 4 5 6 — 02 01 00 99 98 97

To my parents, Lois and Milton Smith, and my siblings,
Dale, Cyndy, Frank, Cecily, and Michelle. May this book
be a blessing to anyone seeking a permanent way
out of endless dieting cycles that can rob them
of the realization of who they are in Christ.

Vivian S. Lamphear, Ph.D.

CONTENTS

WEEK 1

WEEK 2

ACKNOWLEDGMENTS

■ Deep gratitude is expressed to Lois Smith and Cyndy Jaeger for their contributions to the research and preparation of this workbook. A debt of gratitude is owed to James Marlar for his essential computer expertise and the countless hours he contributed to the final preparation process. Thanks, also, to Sandra Jensen, M.S., Craig and Pat Spivack, Greta Sheffer, and Jennifer Cundiff, for the time and effort they gave in the preparation and review of this workbook. We appreciate the support of Brian Hampton and Victor Oliver. Finally, we thank our families for sacrificing their time with us while our efforts were concentrated on the workbook.

INTRODUCTION

by Dr. Vivian Lamphear

■ Readers of our book *Gentle Eating* were excited to learn that gradual, gentle changes in lifestyle and behavior can make weight management permanent and life more enjoyable. We were flooded with requests for a Gentle Eating workbook to provide specific guidelines and practice exercises for lifetime changes. This workbook addresses those requests.

This workbook is based on the successful holistic four STEP plan used by the authors for improved health benefits and permanent weight control:

1. **S = SPIRITUAL**
2. **T = THINKING**
3. **E = EMOTIONAL**
4. **P = PHYSICAL**

The *Gentle Eating Workbook* will

- lead you through a personal journey of self-discovery.
- increase your *spiritual* awareness and growth.
- give you an understanding of how *thinking* influences *emotions* and eating behavior.
- help you develop new behaviors and thinking patterns.
- produce *physical* results that follow naturally from the STEP changes.

There are no quick fixes, magic diets, or promises of a thin body in the *Gentle Eating Workbook*. Its approach differs dramatically from other weight management programs by emphasizing the whole you: spirit, mind, and body.

Following the STEP plan allows you to closely examine how you view yourself and others. You will gain insight into your relationships with others and your current beliefs and myths regarding food, diets, fat, and body appearance. Recognizing and understanding the connections between seemingly unrelated matters will give you new tools to aid you in making healthy changes in your lifestyle. You will learn why and how significant changes from within must precede visible outer changes to assure lasting results.

By incorporating moderate physical activities into your daily routines and understanding your thought processes and emotions, you will automatically give less thought to food and your appearance. You will relearn your healthy childhood behaviors of feeling hunger, meeting your needs, and going on to the next activity.

Relapse prevention is crucial for permanent weight control and is an integral part of the workbook. You will learn how to anticipate and deal with events that may cause you to become sidetracked. Easy-to-follow instructions are provided to identify and change thoughts, feelings, and behaviors that may trigger a cycle of fears including these:

- Gaining weight
- Trying not to eat to avoid overeating
- Becoming more obsessed with food
- Bingeing and overeating

This knowledge will enable you to permanently manage your weight and retain your STEP changes as lifetime commitments for a healthier, happier, more spiritual, and more productive life.

USING THE *GENTLE EATING WORKBOOK*

■ Permanent weight management is a slow, gentle process of transforming Spiritual, Thinking, Emotional, and Physical patterns. The *Gentle Eating Workbook* is your personal guide to exciting STEP changes and is designed for individual or group use. Whatever method you choose, remember this program is for you! You are not competing with anyone; there are no right or wrong answers. Choose your own pace, and proceed toward your goals.

You might find certain sections or exercises in the workbook more relevant than others to your weight loss needs. Feel free to read the chapters in sequence or skip entire sections. As you become more familiar with the STEPs, you may choose to return to portions you have skipped. In fact, many readers reported that they found it useful to go through the workbook several times. Each time they gained new insights and made additional changes.

As you proceed through this workbook, you will find it easier to more completely document your progress. Initially, you may record only information regarding food and physical activity. Later, you may choose to record more detailed information. You might find it beneficial to compile your journal materials in a separate notebook for reviewing and updating your progress. Keep it simple or make it more comprehensive; do what works best for you.

A word about journaling: Journaling or recording your STEP activities is a good way to stay focused and on track with your weight management program. Monitoring your current STEP patterns can act as a springboard for future changes. Being aware of present eating behavior is the first step toward lasting weight management. You might find the "Progress Chart" a useful journaling format. A copy of the chart can be found at the end of each chapter. Alternatively, you may choose your own journaling method.

Do not make journaling a chore! If you do not feel like recording everything every day, then skip it. Your goal is to make the process simple so you will stay with it.

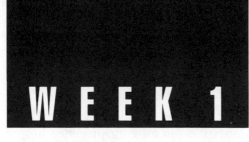

SPIRITUAL:
Understanding Your Relationship with God and Food

■ As long as there is hunger in your soul, a mountain of food will not relieve the emptiness you feel! Only God can fulfill your deepest spiritual and emotional needs. Do you turn to food alone for nourishment, only to find that hunger persists? Turn to God and His Word to understand that as one of His children, you must have sustenance of your soul as well as your body if you are to be healthy and thrive:

> So He humbled you, allowed you to hunger, and fed you with manna
> which you did not know nor did your fathers know, that He might
> make you know that man shall not live by bread alone; but man lives
> by every word that proceeds from the mouth of the LORD (Deut. 8:3).

Connections Between Needs, Unmet Needs, and Food

Everyone has needs that must be met. When you feel your needs are not met on all levels, you are likely to be dissatisfied, confused, and upset. If you resort to abuse of food, your problems will remain unsolved and become magnified. Calm, thoughtful reflection, relying on God's abundant wisdom and strength, will help you form plans to have your needs met. Also, helping others in their times of need will aid you in identifying and solving your difficult situations.

Always remember God is a living presence in your life; walk and talk with Him.

> To You, O my Strength, I will sing praises;
> For God is my defense,
> My God of mercy (Ps. 59:17).

Janet is a forty-one-year-old mother of three who works part-time to keep a step ahead of the bills. After caring for the house, working, attending church activities, and meeting her family's needs, Janet can't imagine having time for herself. In fact, she feels she is on automatic pilot. Her only comfort seems to be food. Janet listed her unmet needs and how she felt she could get them met. At first, Janet thought that such changes were impossible. However, as she thought of creative ways to get her needs met instead of turning to food, the changes followed.

You must give up the myth "you can have and do it all," and you must understand you can't and remain emotionally and physically healthy. Identify and set priorities, then determine what you are willing to give up. Especially, you need to realize constant eating adds to your problems and makes a bad situation much worse:

> Trust in the LORD with all your heart,
> And lean not on your own understanding;
> In all your ways acknowledge Him,
> And He shall direct your paths (Prov. 3:5–6).

EXERCISE

1. Think of needs you feel are unmet. List them.

_____

_____

_____

WEEK 1

2. Do you feel it is possible for these needs to be met? If so, how and by whom?

_____

_____

_____

3. What can you do today to get the process started?

_____

_____

_____

"Abracadabra" Works Only in Fairy Tales

Change is a process that sometimes occurs so slowly, you get impatient. But "presto-chango" and "shazam," like "abracadabra," work only in fairy tales and comic books, and you are living in the real world. Look at sales figures and dollar amounts generated by some of the miracle-promising weight control products on the market today. They're astronomical! No doubt you are familiar with advertisements that state, "Will melt the fat away," "Will prevent the food from turning into fat," "Will cause your body to burn more calories than it takes in," "No need to exercise" (and so on and so forth). And though you know the promises are false, you still harbor some undefined, unfounded hope the creams, salves, lotions, and potions will at least do something. The most you can realistically hope for is that none will harm your body.

Think for a moment: God's Word is filled with proved miracles and fulfilled promises, and you sometimes push that knowledge from your mind. You try expensive products because an aggressive marketing program touts them as cure-alls.

In weight management, what works is slow, gentle lifetime change in your relationships with God and your fellow believers, and your thinking, behavior, and lifestyle. You will learn as you go along what pleases the Lord and be encouraged by the changes you see as you follow the path He has set for you:

The end of a thing is better than its beginning;
The patient in spirit is better than the proud in spirit (Eccl. 7:8).

Have you often heard or said these words: "But I've tried and I can't change"? Take heart! Change is possible. You only have to commit to following the ways of the Lord and doing His will. The changes will come: "If anyone is in Christ, he is a new creation; old things have passed away; behold, all things have become new" (2 Cor. 5:17).

EXERCISE 1

1. Are you impatient for results of change to be immediate?

_____

2. Have you bought and used products that make exaggerated promises you know are false and unrealistic?

_____

3. Think of personal and spiritual changes that will allow you to see results more quickly.

_____

_____

_____

4. What changes do you seek that will require more time?

_____

_____

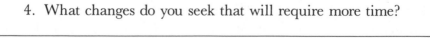

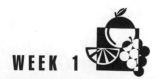

WEEK 1

5. Devise plans for short- and long-term changes you desire so results will be constantly apparent. Make God the firm foundation for all your plans.

_____

_____

6. Think of ways to remind yourself change is a process and takes time.

_____

_____

7. What steps can you take to develop the patience it takes to be gentle with yourself and others?

_____

_____

My brethren, count it all joy when you fall into various trials, knowing that the testing of your faith produces patience. But let patience have its perfect work, that you may be perfect and complete, lacking nothing (James 1:2–4).

EXERCISE 2

1. Whether or not you are aware of it, you have a relationship with God. Study God's Word and become aware of His presence in your life. Learn how a strong loving association with God can help you overcome problems, including food management. Note some points you learn from your Bible study.

_____

_____

And do not seek what you should eat or what you should drink, nor have an anxious mind. For all these things the nations of the world seek after, and your Father knows that you need these things. But seek

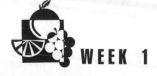

WEEK 1

the kingdom of God, and all these things shall be added to you (Luke 12:29–31).

2. Determine if your food problem is a spiritual problem by asking yourself, Do I attempt to use food to feed a hunger in my life that only a daily association with God can fill?

_____

_____

3. If your answer to the previous question is yes, think of changes you can make that will provide you the fulfillment you seek.

_____

_____

Lord, sometimes familiar things fall away from my life—a move to another city, friends who are now far away, the end of a valued relationship, a change in employment. And with the loss of familiar things, I am confronted with new places, new faces, new challenges. Let me be reminded always that You are the one constant in my life. Help me to avoid sad thoughts, and let me cherish joyful memories. Help me to replace every negative thought with a positive one that will keep me moving toward my goals. Help me to understand that I do not need to turn to food as a comfort, and that I can feel better if I continue to pray for strength and wisdom. Help me to change dark viewpoints into ones illuminated by Your light. Amen.

THINKING:
How Your Thinking Keeps the Weight On

Changing your eating habits and increasing daily physical activities are not enough to keep the weight off. You must also identify and change negative thinking patterns that can trigger overeating. As you

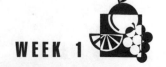

work through the Thinking sections, you will learn how negative thinking styles interfere with weight control success. Distorted thinking styles common to people struggling with food problems are highlighted, and effective ways to develop positive thinking patterns are discussed.

Think Like a Winner While Losing

Negative thinking styles and beliefs related to food and weight control can block your goal to successfully manage your weight. Developing a positive attitude will produce lasting changes in your thought processes and allow you to shed your old ways of thinking and coping. Begin these changes by learning to identify and correct distorted thinking. As your skills increase, you will recognize how feelings of hunger, frustration, the desire to eat, fatigue, and boredom are intertwined.

Studies conducted on the thinking and feelings of overweight individuals treated in a weight loss program in Sweden showed distorted reasoning preceded participants' negative moods, which ultimately led to program failures. Those who were most successful at losing weight reported fewer negative self-statements (e.g., "I'll never lose this weight") or negative feelings (e.g., guilt, depression, low self-worth, anxiety) when they abandoned the diet. The least successful dieters reported numerous negative self-statements and low confidence in their ability to lose weight. People who lost significant amounts of weight did not report feelings of guilt, self-blame, or negative self-statements when they slipped off the diet. Results of the studies suggest thinking has more to do with losing weight and keeping it off than the amount and type of food eaten or the exercise program followed.

Negative emotional states such as anxiety, boredom, and depression make you especially vulnerable to overeating, so you must think positively and build your confidence level. In future chapters, you will learn ways to identify and plan effective responses to difficult or high-risk food situations.

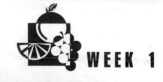

WEEK 1

The Role of Distorted Thinking in Weight Gain

Whether your weight problem is due primarily to medical reasons, inactivity, or overeating, you will learn how your thinking habits can thwart your weight control goal. Thinking errors and distortions that characterize many overeaters appear to keep them in a failure loop, making lasting weight change much harder.

For example, believing weight gain will lead to a miserable life or the loss of love and admiration may cause you to become overly concerned with food and your body size. Focusing on food can lead you to obsess more about it. Feeling fearful you can't control your eating habits may cause you to severely restrict your food intake. And when you tell yourself, "No, I won't eat," you may deprive yourself temporarily but then rebel with a full-blown binge.

Such distorted thinking produces a no-win cycle: fear of weight gain, followed by obsessing about food, deprivation and, ultimately, overeating. This, of course, triggers a fear of weight gain. (See fig. 1.1.) Breaking out of this cycle requires you to (1) recognize and change your erroneous thinking patterns, (2) solve your problems directly, not with food, and (3) return the purpose of food to a physically nourishing role.

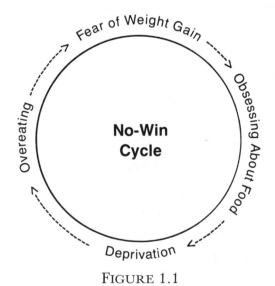

FIGURE 1.1

Healthy eating and weight management do not require willpower. Overeating indicates not a lack of willpower but the result of negative, distorted thinking patterns, which often lead to out-of-control behavior.

Myths and Illogical Thinking Block Permanent Weight Loss

Many overeaters cling to diet myths and superstitions about food and weight. Ironically, this distorted, unrealistic way of thinking often leads to behaviors that actually keep the weight on.

For example, if you step on a scale immediately after breakfast and see more pounds registered than you expected, you may conclude you ate too much and need to skip lunch and dinner to get the weight off. Dieting behavior usually follows, and you skip meals to get the weight off from breakfast, which temporarily reduces your anxiety about gaining weight. Soon, however, the "hunger monster" hovers near, and you look for a quick (usually fattening) way to banish the empty feeling. Attitudes have power; they can help or hurt you.

EXERCISE

Check any of the following comments you have made, and indicate their impact on your eating behavior and weight control efforts:

___ 1. "If I starve or skip meals, I'll lose more weight." (Fact: Metabolism slows down because your body has an instinctive survival mechanism and thinks it is in starvation mode. Skipping meals also leads to a greater preoccupation with food.)

_____

___ 2. "Laxatives, diuretics, and vomiting will speed weight loss." (Fact: While these quick-fix methods of purging temporarily reduce water weight, all three are extremely dangerous and do not result in calorie reductions.)

_____

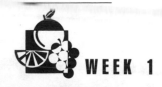 **WEEK 1**

—— 3. "I fail on my diets because I have poor self-control." (Fact: Failure is more likely linked to distorted thinking.)

—— 4. "If I don't lose a lot of weight fast, or if I stop losing weight, the plan isn't working." (Fact: Your body's metabolism may level off if it thinks you are starving. You may need to gently increase exercise to gradually increase metabolism.)

—— 5. "I can sneak these cookies by my body." (Fact: This is a form of denial when you pretend the calorie count automatically goes to zero if you eat quickly or privately. If you indulge in this type of distorted thinking, you believe cutting the size tag out of clothing makes the clothing smaller.)

—— 6. "I'll weigh myself right after overeating to see if I gained any weight." (Fact: Weight gain may take several days to show up on a scale.)

—— 7. "I weigh myself in the morning because I weigh less then." (Fact: This is a meaningless assumption and should not be considered a reliable indicator.)

—— 8. "After I've eaten a lot, I exercise strenuously and then weigh myself to see if I've lost weight." (Fact: You may temporarily lose pounds because of water loss, but lasting weight loss takes time and patience.)

WEEK 1

___ 9. "I rely on a scale to tell me if my program is working." (Fact: Reviewing successes logged in all of the STEP categories provides a better gauge of overall progress than just the number of pounds reflected on a scale.)

_____

Review the exercise, and put a star by the attitudes you are willing to drop.

If you did not place a star next to each attitude, write down reasons why and justify them to yourself.

_____
_____
_____
_____

Keep a Record of Your Self-Talk

Your inner chatter or self-talk can cause you to eat when you're not hungry or binge and overeat by confusing your natural ability to determine true hunger. This inner chatter reflects your beliefs about food, yourself, and unresolved emotional issues. To change self-defeating self-talk, use the following instructions to keep a daily self-talk record:

1. Record what you're saying to yourself. Be patient; it takes a lot of practice to hear your self-talk.

_____
_____

2. Evaluate the truth or validity of what you said (e.g., "I'll never be able to keep this weight off"). What concrete, objective evidence do you have that the statement is true?

_____
_____

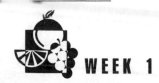

WEEK 1

3. Record how your thoughts make you feel.

_____

_____

4. Record a more appropriate or valid statement regarding your thoughts, feelings, or behavior.

_____

_____

EMOTIONAL:
Recognizing the Source of Your Emotions

Though events may appear to cause your emotions (e.g., someone makes a disparaging remark and you become angered or depressed), your emotions are determined not by the event itself but by your interpretation of the event: what the event means to you. Your view of yourself and the world defines your expectations and the meanings events have for you.

You cannot always change events, but you can change how you think about them. Specifically, you can reevaluate your expectations and the meanings you attach to events. The following example illustrates how the way you think about an event determines your moods and feelings.

Yvonne's husband remarked about her eating behavior, "Are you going to eat that?" She thought to herself, *He thinks I'm a worthless pig. He's right. I always eat too much.* This negative thought led to immediate feelings of hopelessness, depression, and anger. Yvonne responded by eating the "whole thing, just to show him." Later, she reflected on what her husband said. Feeling depressed again, she consumed a large bowl of ice cream to ease her pain.

A comment by Yvonne's husband triggered her distorted thinking. She labeled herself a "worthless pig," which caused her to feel angry and depressed. Yvonne made three thinking errors that resulted in her feelings of discouragement and ultimately led to her overeating binge.

First, she engaged in mind reading. Without clarifying what her husband meant, Yvonne assumed he thought she was a "worthless pig." That is certainly enough to make her feel down about herself!

Second, referring to herself as a "worthless pig" is known as labeling. When she negatively labeled herself, she evaluated her total worth in terms of one supposed negative quality.

Third, Yvonne overgeneralized when she said, "I always eat too much." This thought or belief led to feelings of despair about her ability to change her eating behavior. Her feeling of hopelessness resulted in her using food as a comfort rather than dealing with the situation directly.

Perhaps you recognize this familiar pattern: Something is said or happens, and you interpret it in a certain way, which is then reflected in your self-talk. Negative or distorted thinking leads to negative, discouraging feelings, which often influence your eating behavior.

You may be tempted to use food as an anodyne after experiencing negative emotions. Eating will likely distract you and make you feel better for a while; however, you may later experience guilt, anxiety, or depression over your actions. The self-defeating cycle of negative thinking, negative feelings, and overeating then continues and explains why you may find it difficult to keep weight off.

Had Yvonne identified and challenged her negative self-talk, the emotional outcome might have been different. She could have interpreted the same event in a more objective way by thinking, *That's a rude remark. My weight program is* my *business. I've been doing well in general.* An assertive response to her husband could have been: "I appreciate your concern about my weight, but I feel that remark is a put-down. I need your positive comments to acknowledge and encourage my commitment to my program. Please do not make negative remarks to me."

WEEK 1

Formats and instructions for keeping a journal and progress chart are provided in this workbook. If Yvonne had been keeping a progress chart, she would have noted that she handled a difficult situation in a positive way. She would have been able to see that she is learning to be more assertive, and reviewing her progress might have been enough to encourage her to stay on track. Finally, instead of turning to food when she felt an impulse to eat, she might have sipped a favorite beverage or glass of water, called a friend to chat on the telephone, or taken a brief walk.

Change Your Thinking to Change Your Feelings

The first step in changing automatic negative thoughts is to identify them. Next, notice the feelings that follow the thoughts. Then, reevaluate your expectations (e.g., husbands should always say encouraging things) and the meaning the event has for you (e.g., one slip on the program means your efforts are useless and your situation is hopeless). The reevaluation of the event should be objective and realistic. Finally, record how you feel after reevaluating the event.

Following is an exercise format you can use to practice changing thoughts that can lead to negative emotions. As you record your thoughts, notice how difficult they are to identify and change. That is because they are so ingrained into your belief system. But with practice, you will learn to recognize and change automatic negative thoughts. Sometimes it is easier to record the feeling first and then work backward to record the distortion. Use the method that works best for you.

EXERCISE

1. Record negative thoughts.

_____

_____

_____

_____

WEEK 1

2. Record feelings that follow the thoughts.

_____

_____

_____

_____

3. Reevaluate your self-talk.

_____

_____

_____

_____

4. Record any changes in your feelings.

_____

_____

_____

Emotional Eating

Instead of dealing directly with an event, stress, or problem at hand, many overweight people resort to eating as a solution or diversion. This is classified as emotional eating. Though overeating is a problem for both men and women, according to an article in *Family Circle* (June 8, 1993), "women are twice as likely to rely on food to feel better when they are depressed."

As you progress in your program, you will learn to recognize how negative and distorted thinking can lead to feelings of anxiety, depression, and anger, which may trigger emotional eating. Also, you will learn how to develop specific strategies to identify and change patterns of behavior that precede, accompany, or follow such binges.

Defining Depression

Listed below are the classic symptoms of depression as defined by the American Psychiatric Association:

WEEK 1

___ 1. Noticeable change of appetite or sleeping patterns
___ 2. Loss of interest in activities previously enjoyed
___ 3. Fatigue; loss of energy
___ 4. Feelings of worthlessness and hopelessness
___ 5. Feelings of inappropriate guilt
___ 6. Inability to concentrate or think; indecisiveness
___ 7. Recurring thoughts of death or suicide
___ 8. Overwhelming feelings of sadness and grief
___ 9. Headaches or stomachaches

If you have four or more of these symptoms for more than two weeks, you are advised to seek help.

Check any of the above symptoms that you feel apply to you.

Can you trace the origins of any symptoms you checked?

_____
_____
_____
_____

If you feel you are suffering from depression and the condition is not temporary, make appropriate decisions regarding treatment.

_____
_____

EXERCISE

1. What emotions tempt you to eat/overeat?

_____
_____

2. What/who triggers these emotions?

_____
_____

Why Compulsive Overeating?

Although many people who struggle with weight management recall a happy childhood, others relate their food problems to some form of unresolved childhood pain or unmet needs. Never learning healthier ways to cope, some began relying on food in reaction to stress, depression, anger, anxiety, fear, and/or hurt.

You may feel a sense of temporary relief from emotional stress when you behave compulsively, either by overeating or by giving in to other addictions. Such behavior may appear to immediately meet your most basic physical and emotional needs. However, this temporary relief is often followed by feelings of shame, guilt, and depression. Lasting change can occur only if you recognize when, how, and why you resort to self-defeating behavior and take positive steps to eliminate the causes.

EXERCISE

1. Has eating and/or food become a compulsive addiction for you?

_____

2. If you answered yes, describe how and why you think the problem developed.

_____

_____

3. How do you rely on food to cope with past or present pain?

_____

_____

4. How does food help you get through the day?

_____

_____

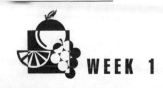

WEEK 1

5. Do you rely on food to deal with stress? In what ways?

PHYSICAL:
"Getting Physical" with Food, Weight, and Body Image

Read each question and circle yes or no.

YES NO   1. Am I overly concerned and preoccupied with food?

YES NO   2. Am I overly concerned and preoccupied with how much I weigh?

YES NO   3. Am I overly concerned with and distressed by my body shape?

YES NO   4. Do my weight and body shape determine my self-worth?

YES NO   5. Is achieving thinness more important to me than just about anything?

YES NO   6. Do I feel thinness equals happiness?

YES NO   7. Do I feel being overweight means I am a failure or loser?

YES NO   8. Do I think I have the ability to change my eating habits?

YES NO   9. Are there times when I refuse to eat at all?

YES NO 10. Do I eat primarily diet or nonfat foods?

YES NO 11. Do I rely on laxatives, diuretics, or purging to control my weight?

YES NO 12. Do I hate the way my body looks?

YES NO 13. Does my self-esteem go up and down as my weight does?

YES NO 14. Do I compare my size and shape to those of people around me?

YES NO 15. Do I feel instantly depressed when the scale shows I've gained weight?

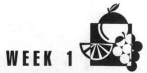

YES NO   16. Do I look in the mirror several times daily to check how my body looks?

Answering yes to three or more questions indicates you may be making unhealthy food choices or have a problem with weight management. Suggestions for gentle, gradual changes to achieve permanent weight control and enjoy a healthier lifestyle are provided in this workbook.

A Simple Equation

Losing or gaining weight is an equation of calories eaten and calories burned, taking into consideration which calories not immediately used by your body are stored as fat and which are flushed from your system. However, calories from fats, carbohydrates, and proteins have definite health benefits, and they are processed differently as you will learn.

Why Traditional Dieting Does Not Work

Continuing studies show the success rate of most diets to be dismal at best. Estimates are that only 5 to 10 percent of overweight individuals maintain a weight loss of twenty pounds or more longer than two years. For this reason, weight loss centers cater to many repeat customers.

A common belief is that poor self-control and lack of willpower are responsible for unsuccessful weight control. This belief fosters feelings of low self-worth, depression, and overeating and is, in fact, untrue. Numerous factors influence eating patterns, some of which we have already addressed. As you learn more about these dietary influences and the difference in self-control and willpower, you will be better prepared to plan your weight management program.

Chronic dieters generally restrict both the quantity and the type of food they consume, hoping to achieve thinness or avoid fatness. Consequently, they often skip entire meals. When they eat meals, the type of food they select is usually labeled low calorie. Often the dieters begin the day with a strong resolve to consume less food, but as the

WEEK 1

day progresses, mounting hunger and food cravings lead to increased awareness of food.

Preoccupied with thoughts of food and eating, chronic dieters may have difficulty focusing on daily activities. This type of behavior can lead to uncontrolled eating, and undereating and overeating may become habitual. Nutritional deprivation often results, and chronic dieters may not understand the serious nature and consequences of this behavior.

Diet Thinking

1. There is an initial psyching up or mental preparedness. The illusion of willpower increases. There is a "high" connected to the feeling of power at the thought of being thin.

2. Food obsessions (in the forms of bingeing, restricting, deprivation, purging, dieting) dominate each day. Excessive time is spent in special preparations and menu planning. Food is the primary focus of each day. There is an emotional high at being in control.

3. The end of the diet is the primary goal. The future (how many pounds more to go) dictates the time frame.

4. As the diet progresses, anxiety increases as the illusion of willpower decreases.

5. Thoughts toward the end of the diet dwell on what we again can eat that we were deprived of when dieting. Food fantasies increase. Cheating and sneaking "forbidden" foods often occur. Guilt over the deception and loss of control increases.

6. When the diet ends, we are no better off than before, for our thin bodies are doomed to relapse. Moreover, our "willpower" will be weaker with subsequent efforts. Physically, our metabolism is negatively altered. Emotionally, we feel defeated. Spiritually, we feel empty.

7. A diet's structure crumbles, as do our efforts. Even so, a false sense of pride and control is projected.

8. A diet results in lowered self-esteem and self-deprecating thoughts and feelings.

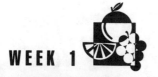

Keeping a Food Diary

Are you a grazer, always eating a little of this and a little of that? Can you recognize other eating habits that sidetrack your resolve to eat healthier? The purpose of a food diary is to make you aware of types and amounts of food you eat each day. This is a first step to accountability for your eating patterns and an understanding of why you eat as you do.

Researchers have found that one reason excess weight seems so hard to shed is that many of us eat more food than we remember—perhaps as much as one thousand calories more per day. Before you say, "One thousand calories a day! No way! I would certainly notice that many extra calories!" commit to keeping a food diary.

Participants in Johns Hopkins University's Health, Weight, and Stress Program are directed to keep a food consumption diary and review it nightly. "We find that most people start losing even before they've begun to diet, because the diary makes them conscious of eating patterns," says program director Maria Simonson, M.D. She advises that entries be logged in right away because if you wait, you tend to forget.

Instructions for Food Diary

At least for a few days, keep a food diary and write down everything you eat. Record significant persons, triggers, and feelings. Include small tastes and samples; they have calories, too. Research has suggested that overweight people tend to forget some of the food they eat, particularly snacks. The food diary is not meant to make you feel guilty; rather, it will allow you to learn more about your eating habits and how you can change them to achieve your goals.

You might carry a notepad and pen to record everything you eat as soon as possible. Later, you can transfer the notes to your Food Diary Chart to allow you an overview at week's end.

WEEK 1

If you would feel more comfortable, keep your chart private. However, studies have indicated that being open and honest can keep you responsible and accountable. Sharing may allow you to come up with alternative activities to eating when you first feel hunger pangs and provide other benefits as well. You know what is best for you, so let the choice be yours.

Continuing a diary may seem burdensome to you, but try to document enough information to evaluate your eating patterns and initiate changes you feel are needed. Try to determine the following:

- Hunger level using 0–10 rating scale: 0 = starved, 5 = satisfied, and 10 = stuffed
- Times of day you usually schedule meals
- Where you eat (home, work, school, car, mall)
- Other people usually present
- Typical thoughts you have before, during, and after meals
- Emotional triggers influencing your overeating

(You can use the format provided on page 23 for keeping your Daily Food Diary Chart or design one of your own.)

EXERCISE

Problem	Possible Solution
1. Preparing meals, snacks, and desserts, and I sample.	
2. Sitting at a meeting and food is present; I snack.	
3. Food is left on the table, and I take a little more.	

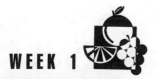

WEEK 1

22

DAILY FOOD DIARY CHART

	MON.	TUES.	WED.	THURS.	FRI.	SAT.	SUN.
1. RATE HUNGER LEVEL							
2. TIME OF DAY							
3. LOCATION (WHERE YOU ATE)							
4. WHO WAS PRESENT							
5. THOUGHTS/ FEELINGS BEFORE/ DURING/ AFTER EATING							
6. EMOTIONAL TRIGGERS FOR OVEREATING							
7. FOODS AND AMOUNTS EATEN							

Small Changes, Big Dividends

Weight loss programs traditionally use number of pounds lost or gained as the primary indicator of success or failure. That limited measure cannot reflect the daily progress you make in each STEP area and may give more importance to a slip than it deserves. Focusing solely on weight also creates illogical and obsessive behaviors that could lead to weight gain.

Lasting change results from gradual, gentle progress in each of the STEP areas. Eating certain foods, limiting others, and experiencing fluctuating weight gain are small parts of the whole picture. Instead of encouraging a limited view of progress (for example, relying on numbers on a scale), you will learn to record and evaluate several different indicators of program success.

Use the following guidelines to chart your progress.

PROGRESS CHART

Check all that apply.

Spiritual Changes

— Had at least a fifteen-minute daily quiet time.

— Memorized a Bible verse.

— Met with midweek church group.

— Went to church services.

— Prayed.

— Felt a little closer to the Lord.

— Expressed true feelings to God.

— Honestly evaluated my relationship with God.

Thinking Changes

— Recognized and recorded a distorted thought.

— Experienced change in how I view myself.

— Experienced change in how I thought about a situation.

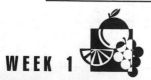

WEEK 1

PROGRESS CHART

Check all that apply.

___ Was able to develop more accurate/balanced view of person, event, etc.

Emotional Changes

___ Recorded my feelings.

___ Evaluated feelings before eating.

___ Expressed feelings in appropriate manner.

___ Noticed impact a person, place, or event had on my urge to eat.

___ Identified a past trauma or hurt.

___ Sought support from a trusted person.

___ Expressed hurt or pain in appropriate way.

___ Noticed how past hurt was related to urge to eat.

___ Worked on a stage of grief.

___ Noticed a change in level of a negative emotion.

___ Noticed a different reaction to person, place, or event that used to evoke emotional upset.

___ Implemented clear, personal emotional boundaries.

Physical/Behavioral Changes

___ Charted my eating patterns.

___ Did workbook exercises.

___ Tried a new low-fat recipe.

___ Performed at least ten minutes of physical activity.

___ Listened to or watched ten to twenty minutes of a relaxation tape (audio or video).

___ Took at least fifteen minutes for myself.

___ Left some food on my plate.

___ Set a nice table with special touches: flowers, tablecloth, candles; listened to soothing music during mealtime; used special dishes.

___ Went shopping when not hungry.

___ Ate intended portions and stopped.

___ Rated hunger level before and after meals.

WEEK 1

Exploring the Roots of Your Eating Habits

Overeating is perhaps the most common cause of weight gain. While overeating may be triggered by a stressful or emotional event, the seriousness and duration of the problem are influenced by individual, family, and societal factors.

Individual Factors

Genetics (heredity) lays the framework for your body's development. Recent research has shown the number and size of fat cells and metabolism are genetically determined. You may ask, "Does that mean I have no control over the matter, and my desire for permanent weight management is futile?" Definitely not. But you need to be knowledgeable and realistic about what your ideal healthy weight can be.

Studies are ongoing, but there are indications chronic yo-yo (lose, gain) dieting may cause rapid weight gain after rapid weight loss. This tendency further enforces the importance of a plan to guide you to balanced, steady, nonextreme Gentle Eating.

Research suggests the yo-yo syndrome may alter metabolism, making it more difficult to lose weight and keep it off each successive time. There is no conclusive evidence, but repeated metabolic changes do appear to raise blood pressure and the ratio of fat to muscle. The need to follow a gentle weight management program as part of your daily routine is clear and may prevent you from compromising your health.

Metabolism: Keeping the Calories Burning

The human body has been compared to, or referred to as, a highly efficient engine, and of course, an engine requires fuel. Steadily putting small amounts of healthy food into your body throughout the day keeps the calories burning efficiently, metabolizing them into energy at a steady pace.

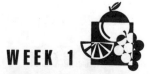

Skipping meals causes your metabolism to slow down, conserving energy. When you finally eat, especially if you overeat, it is more difficult for your body to speed up to burn calories. During this catch-up period, your energy level is lowered, and you may feel fatigued. Avoid low-energy periods by planning mealtimes at regular intervals.

Another advantage of eating several small meals daily is that your body can predict it will be fed and fear of deprivation is eliminated. When your body knows it will stay refueled, overeating is less likely. Your hunger signals become insistent for a quick fix when you go for long periods of time without food. Keeping your blood sugar level steady can prevent a red alert response to your appetite's signal for high-fat and/or high-sugar foods.

Increase Number of Daily Meals, Not Calories

Consider some suggestions to raise your metabolic rate and burn more calories.

Keep those calories burning! Eat small amounts of fruits, vegetables, rice cakes, or other healthy snacks throughout the day to keep your metabolism moving at an even pace and your blood sugar level constant.

Eat carbohydrates to keep your metabolic rate up. Eating fruits, whole grains, and vegetables before your main meal signals to your brain that you are less hungry and you will likely eat less. Studies have indicated that during digestion, 25 percent of the calories from carbohydrates are burned, whereas only 3 percent of fat calories are burned. Remaining calories are stored as fat.

Avoid eating large meals. When you eat big meals, your blood sugar level rises, less fat is burned, and fat storage is triggered.

Drink at least eight eight-ounce containers of water daily. Sipping water throughout the day should become a lifelong habit. When you drink sufficient amounts of water, body fat is burned, stored water is released, and toxins and waste materials are flushed from your body.

WEEK 1

Eat foods rich in iodine. Fish is high in iodine and aids the body's production of thyroxine. Thyroxine is produced by the thyroid gland and is essential in the regulation of metabolism.

Keep on the move. Physical activity that elevates your heart rate increases your metabolism and burns fat. Engage in a physical activity you enjoy for about forty minutes daily at least four days a week. The workout periods may be broken down into ten- or fifteen-minute sessions if they are easier to schedule, but the goal is approximately forty minutes daily. It is generally believed that after twenty minutes, your heart rate is sufficiently high to burn fat, but studies have shown that mini-workouts are also beneficial.

Lift (moderate size) weights. Adopt a gentle, consistent weight-lifting program to build muscles and expend energy, resulting in a leaner body mass. For women, lifting lighter weights can give the desired result without the muscle bulk. Do not overdo!

Eat spices. Jalapeno peppers, chilies, and cinnamon, among other spices, speed up your metabolism. Add spices to your daily meals for improved taste and health benefits.

The Fate of Your Weight: A Fat Gene

Does a "fat gene" determine your metabolic rate and affix your permanent weight? An article published in the *New England Journal of Medicine* suggests if you are overweight, your metabolism works against you when you try to maintain weight loss. This notion is related to the set point theory, which proposes your body reacts to maintain a certain weight level. Your set point is thought to be genetically influenced.

Set point theory indicates your brain resists weight change by sending signals affecting your hunger level, physical activity, and metabolism. According to this theory, your set point is partially determined by what could be described as a biological thermostat.

A number of factors such as stress levels, age, cigarette smoking, and exercise appear to influence the set point, but it appears to be

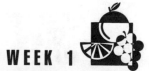

more flexible during adolescence and pregnancy. Set point theory could explain why most dieters fail to keep weight off and, why some people can eat lots of food without gaining weight.

By following the Gentle Eating plan and engaging in daily non-stressful physical activities, you can alter your metabolic set point. You can ask your physician to measure your metabolism rate if you are interested in that information.

EXERCISE 1

1. Have you used the "my metabolism is too slow" excuse to delay a weight management program? Do you believe that exercising is a waste of time? Does your attitude block your progress?

_____

_____

_____

2. If you answered yes to the above questions, list ways you can change your attitude.

_____

_____

_____

3. List several gentle exercise routines you would be willing to try for a few days. Then note differences, if any, in blood circulation and energy level. Even in such a short time, there should be beneficial changes to motivate you to continue exercising. ("Slow and easy" will prevent exercise fatigue and burnout.)

_____

_____

_____

_____

_____

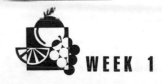

WEEK 1

EXERCISE 2

The set point theory appears to have merit, but you still hold the following beliefs about weight management. Circle yes or no.

YES NO 1. I have a slow metabolism.

YES NO 2. I have tried normal eating and I can't do it.

YES NO 3. I will probably always have to go on diets from time to time.

YES NO 4. I cannot overcome my slow metabolism no matter what I do.

EXERCISE 3

If you answered yes to any of the above questions, what evidence do you require to change those beliefs?

_____

_____

_____

_____

_____

_____

Other Considerations

Other individual factors associated with your eating habits could include low self-esteem, difficulty with autonomy, need to control, and perfectionism. For persons with eating disorders, self-esteem fluctuates with weight and shape.

Anorexia and bulimia are serious eating disorders perhaps suffered by only a small fraction, if any, of this workbook's users. However, statistics show that anorexia and bulimia affect more individuals in the U.S. and other countries than researchers previously thought. It may prove beneficial for you to be aware of some of the symptoms and

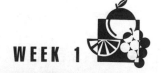

consequences of these disorders. (A cautionary note: These diseases are always best dealt with in professional circumstances.)

Anorexics and bulimics often grow up in chaotic families or have parents or caregivers with exceptionally high standards. Yet, it appears they have problems separating from their parents or caregivers and family. Weight loss, purging, and deprivation are considered tangible means of control over the family's emotional and lifestyle chaos.

Body weight becomes a significant source of self-control and personal identification. Rather than face daily problems directly, the anorexic and the bulimic turn the focus toward weight and weight loss.

EXERCISE 1

1. Which, if any, of the above individual factors pertain to you?

_____

_____

_____

2. How, if at all, do these individual factors relate to your problem with food?

_____

_____

_____

EXERCISE 2

Complete the following weight management readiness inventory. Circle yes or no.

YES NO 1. The thought of changing my relationship with food seems overwhelming.

YES NO 2. I feel everything must be in order before I can make changes in my relationship with food.

WEEK 1

YES NO 3. I don't think I can keep the weight off. I have tried a hundred times before.

YES NO 4. I'm not ready for the reaction I get from others when I reveal my ideal size.

Review your answers and determine what issues are blocking your weight management plan. List ways to resolve these issues.

_____

_____

_____

How Behavior Keeps Weight On

Dieting is the most common form of weight control among individuals seeking to shed unwanted pounds. Often a dieter skips meals, drastically reduces food portions, and avoids foods considered fattening. Many diets require restrictions of food intake far below what the body demands for healthy functioning. When food deprivation is severe enough, the body taps into its stored fat supply to make up the energy deficit, and weight drops.

Overeating can be a consequence of caloric deprivation, and what started out as a measure to reduce weight becomes a trigger that produces self-defeating behavior. Following prolonged intake restriction, the body craves high-fat and salty foods to quickly restore a depleted fat supply. Dieting, usually followed by bingeing, may result in an unhealthy cycle and may lead to dangerous habits of self-induced vomiting and the abuse of laxatives and diuretics.

Binge Eating. An episode of eating in which an excessive amount of food is consumed in an uncontrolled manner is commonly referred to as binge eating. It typically involves a strong craving for high-calorie carbohydrates and fats, coupled with feelings of anxiety, depression, frustration, or boredom. These moods may be the result of any unpleasant emotional experience or constant stress.

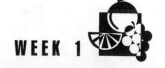

WEEK 1

The speed of eating and type and quantity of food eaten are experienced as beyond the person's control. Usually done in secrecy, the binge ends only at the point the person runs out of food, is interrupted by others, or becomes painfully full. Afterward, the person may suffer abdominal pain with bloating as well as feelings of self-disgust, guilt, or anxiety about possible weight gain. During a binge, the person is distracted from unpleasant thoughts or feelings, but they invariably return when the episode has ended.

Self-Induced Vomiting. This destructive behavior is often used by persons wanting to prevent the effect of calories ingested during a binge episode. The binge-vomiting cycle usually escalates over time. Eventually, bingers may feel compelled to vomit anytime food believed to lead to weight gain is ingested.

Vomiting causes electrolyte disturbances in the body that can pose serious health risks, such as injuries to the heart. Prolonged bingeing and purging also lead to esophagus damage and dental problems. Even temporary weight loss achieved by this method is highly detrimental to physical and emotional health.

Laxatives and Diuretics. The use of laxatives and diuretics is not only ineffective for permanent weight loss, but also dangerous to the body's systems. Laxatives empty the large intestine after calories have been absorbed in the small intestine, and diuretics only temporarily rid the body of water. Prolonged dependence on diuretics can cause serious dehydration and produce electrolyte imbalance.

When the body is dehydrated, its reaction is to store and retain water, which registers as a weight gain on a scale. Contrary to what many chronic dieters believe, increasing the daily water intake lowers excessive water retention, facilitates metabolic processes, and serves as an appetite suppressant.

Physical Exercise. Moderate exercise benefits the body in numerous ways. It builds muscle, which burns more fat, speeds up metabolism, lowers blood pressure, and speeds up the cardiovascular system.

WEEK 1

However, the focus of strenuous exercising is often to burn unwanted calories, especially right after a meal. Strenuous exercise never fully compensates for a decreased metabolic rate caused by excessive dieting but reflects the person is still in a binge-purge mode.

One important step of the Gentle Eating plan is moderate daily exercise. Avoid exercise regimens that are too vigorous.

Excessive Scale Weighing. Do you go through phases when you obsessively weigh on a scale several times a day, allowing the scale to determine not only how you eat, but also how you feel and behave? The scale reflects a number you like and you feel happy. If not, you are likely depressed and anxious. Relying on a scale to reflect weight control progress also sets you up for illogical behavior in your eating and exercising habits. Do not allow a scale to do your thinking for you!

Other Behaviors That Keep the Weight On. Obvious behaviors that keep weight on include being sedentary most of the day, not pushing away from the table soon enough, and not performing daily physical activity or exercise.

EXERCISE

1. Do you engage in any of the behaviors noted above?

_____

2. Is your inability to control your weight linked to these behaviors? How?

_____

_____

_____

3. List ways to avoid the behaviors.

_____

_____

_____

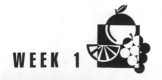

WEEK 1

Family Factors

Family factors can interact with individual and societal variables to influence weight management. Attitudes toward the body weights and shapes of both men and women are often transmitted by significant family members, especially parents or caregivers. Remarks made by family members regarding food and exercise habits may intimidate others in the family. Additional family characteristics that may be related to development of eating problems include the following:

__ Inability to resolve conflicts

__ Overly protective parents or caregivers

__ Overly critical parents or caregivers

__ Parents or caregivers expecting perfection or having exceptionally high standards

__ Overly rigid house rules

__ Unclear family boundaries (roles reversed)

__ Family history of depression or alcoholism

__ History of sexual or physical abuse

EXERCISE

1. Check any of the above factors you have experienced.

2. How do you think these factors may relate to your weight problem?

_____

_____

Societal Factors

In the U.S., thin men and women are often portrayed as being happier, more sophisticated, better at their careers, more socially successful, and generally leading better lives. Being thin does not ensure physical fitness, but many men and women tend to determine their

WEEK 1

self-worth according to body weight and shape. Therefore, their self-worth rises or plummets as their weight and shape fluctuate.

Frequently, magazine surveys ask readers to answer the question "What would make you happiest?" Survey results show most respondents put weight loss at the top of their list with success at work usually ranking second. Further, researchers gathered numerous answers to one query, "What is it that you want to stop doing?" They then listed in order items that people said gave them the most trouble when they tried to quit. Number one was overeating (*Orange County Register,* December 4, 1995).

Often, men and women want their bodies to match the unrealistic ideals portrayed in the media, and when they do not measure up, they believe it is their fault. Commercials bombard viewers with visions of irresistible, delectable foods, then the next frame or sentence implies, "You are desirable only if you are thin." Conflicting messages of "eat" and "do not eat" are flashed to the brain, laying the groundwork for potential eating problems.

You do not expect everyone to have the same shoe size or be the same height, so why should everyone strive to weigh the same according to arbitrary rules involving gender, age, and height? Such aspirations are unrealistic, and charts reciting such information should serve as a general reference only.

WEEK 2

SPIRITUAL:
Learning to Stay
the Course

■ Some situations in which you find yourself may prompt you to ask, Why did God allow this to happen to me? Do you stay angry about the life God gave you and doubt His love for you?

Recall that Job faced incredible pain, suffering, and loss that seemed unjust and unfair to him. Why God would put him through such misery was beyond his comprehension. Nevertheless, through all his anger and confusion about God's motives or plan for his life, Job maintained his faith in the Lord: "And the LORD restored Job's losses when he prayed for his friends. Indeed the LORD gave Job twice as much as he had before" (Job 42:10).

God is constantly with you through both good and bad times; lean on Him. In your way of thinking, suffering and pain are experiences to be avoided, but God uses your anguish and trials to further mold you. Learn more about your relationship with God, and though at times it may be difficult to understand, know God is working His good in your life according to His plan.

EXERCISE

1. Read Romans 5:1–5; Job 42:1–5; and James 1:2–4. In what ways do these passages relate to situations in your life?

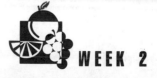

_____

_____

2. Do you let uncontrolled anger affect your relationship with God and others?

_____

_____

3. God is constantly with you; call on His wisdom and strength in your times of need, and record what happens.

_____

_____

4. Trust and obey Him in all things. Through prayer and the reading of His Word, what have you learned about His many promises to you and what is required of you in the keeping of those promises?

_____

_____

_____

5. Developing a persistent faith is gradual. Be patient. Be gentle. Make notes to yourself about how your faith is developing.

_____

_____

_____

Lord, it is with a grateful heart that I come to You in prayer. I have delighted in this day and my walks and talks with You. Thank You for all the blessings You have given me. Help me to be ever mindful that just as my earthly body must have sustenance, so do my soul and spirit. Stay by my side, and help me become healthier and stronger in spirit, mind, and body. I am Your servant in all things, Lord, and I have placed my life in Your loving hands. Amen.

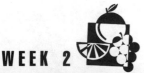

WEEK 2

Knowing God; Knowing Yourself

You are created in the image of God; therefore, you must truly come to know God to know yourself. When Jesus was asked, "Which is the first commandment of all?" He answered in Mark 12:29–30: "The first of all the commandments is: 'Hear, O Israel, the LORD our God, the LORD is one. And you shall love the LORD your God with all your heart, with all your soul, with all your mind, and with all your strength.' This is the first commandment." He then added in verse 31: "And the second, like it, is this: 'You shall love your neighbor as yourself.' There is no other commandment greater than these." Like the loving Father He is, He is letting you know what He expects and requires of you.

In God's eyes, a career, financial success, and an education mean nothing if you fail to develop a close and loving relationship with Him and your neighbors. But, you might ask yourself, doesn't He know that it is sometimes difficult for me to understand and tolerate some of the people in my life, much less love them? You, of course, know the answer to that question: Yes, He does know. That is exactly why He gave such importance to the commandment; He wanted you to have no room for doubt. Your meaning and purpose in life are set forth: Love God; love others. Jesus said, "A new commandment I give to you, that you love one another; as I have loved you, that you also love one another. By this all will know that you are My disciples, if you have love for one another" (John 13:34–35).

EXERCISE 1

1. Through His Word and prayer, get to know God better. Begin this very day! David wrote,

> Behold, how good and how pleasant it is
> For brethren to dwell together in unity! (Ps. 133:1).

 **WEEK 2**

Note some things you've learned about God.

_____

_____

2. As you strengthen your relationship with God and better understand God and yourself, think of gentle ways to express your love through words and deeds.

_____

_____

3. Do you find losing your fear or reluctance to express or accept warm feelings makes it easier to love others? How?

_____

_____

4. Do you blame God or others for your problems?

_____

As you learn more about your relationship with God and others, and as your thinking becomes more clear, do you find the blame was misplaced?

_____

_____

_____

5. Have you been waiting to receive God's grace and love until your problems were solved and you felt worthy? Does this thinking delay or prohibit your spiritual growth and block attainment of your goals? How?

_____

_____

_____

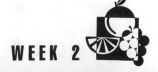

Let us therefore come boldly to the throne of grace, that we may
obtain mercy and find grace to help in time of need (Heb. 4:16).

6. Are you so consumed with thoughts of your struggles and food
that you leave no room for God or anyone or anything else? Change
your thoughts, and with God's help your strength will be renewed and
your life's journey will be a happier one. Realize you do not have to
trudge on alone. God is always by your side; turn to Him and know
Him as a loving companion. He will not fail you! Write your thoughts
on this subject.

_____

_____

God is our refuge and strength,
A very present help in trouble (Ps. 46:1).

EXERCISE 2

1. In the past I felt unworthy to receive God's love or the love of
others because

_____

2. In a sense, do I feel I might have allowed food to become more
important than God in my life? In what way?

_____

3. I sometimes feel God has abandoned me because

_____

4. What is my image of God? What do I expect of Him?

_____

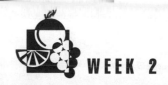

5. With a better understanding of God and after studying His stated expectations and requirements of me, are my image and expectations of Him realistic? Have I changed my thinking? How?

_____

_____

6. If my thinking has changed, am I less confused and better able to pursue my goals? In what way?

_____

_____

7. Have I given the church a chance to be a part of my spiritual life? Do I feel the church has failed me? In what way or ways? What do I feel the church has to offer me?

_____

_____

_____

THINKING:
Stop the Flow of Negative Thoughts

Depressed individuals are likely to arrive at incorrect conclusions about themselves, others, and their world by making false assumptions. They often see things in black and white and view themselves and their behavior in a mostly negative light. Their positive qualities and behaviors are often minimized or discounted. Labeling themselves in general negative terms (for example, "I'm just a lazy slob") perpetuates feelings of hopelessness and despair. Similar distorted thinking patterns that can lead to feelings of depression, anxiety, and low self-confidence are exhibited by many overeaters. During the next few weeks, you will continue to learn and practice how to identify, record, challenge, and change thinking patterns that interfere with your weight management program. As your efforts are rewarded by positive thoughts and actions, you will feel a higher level of self-confidence and recognize your path to success is smoother. Make this a goal: Anxiety and depression will have to find a new place to dwell; your mind will no longer be their home. Always think like a winner!

Challenge Your Negative Thinking

An effective method for identifying and changing your distorted thinking is keeping a Thought Record to help you view any lapses or slips in your program in a less emotional way (see fig. 2.1). Changing your negative thinking will make gaining control over your eating habits easier. You can quickly implement corrections rather than spiral downward in a negative flow of self-blame, guilt, and continued over-eating.

Using a four-column format, in the first column give a brief description of the triggers for overeating. Use the second column to record your thoughts during and after the episode, and the third column to identify particular thinking distortions. In the fourth column, reevaluate your self-statements. Try to be objective and balanced in reviewing what happened and determining the impact on you.

All or None Thinking

All or none thinking occurs when you see things in black and white categories. Perfectionism is the basis of all or none thinking, and less-than-perfect control at all times is construed as total failure. For example, you overeat one time and are sure you lack willpower and will never manage your weight. There is no middle ground or gray area to foster belief that once a slip has occurred, you can employ coping measures and stay on the path to success

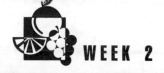

WEEK 2

THOUGHT RECORD

TRIGGERS: Briefly describe event leading to overeating	THOUGHTS: Record automatic thoughts that accompany behavior	THINKING DISTORTIONS: Identify distortions present in each automatic thought	REEVALUATION OF SELF-STATEMENTS: Record coping responses to automatic thoughts
Example: Ate appropriately at breakfast, but ate too much at lunch following stressful morning.	"I can't believe I ate all that. I have no willpower and will never lose weight! I'm a total failure at changing my eating behavior."	All or none thinking Labeling Overgeneralization	"I'm not a totally successful weight manager, but I am making progress. This is one event; I slipped. I can choose what I will do next time."
Overate at dinner because I was depressed about stuffing myself at lunch. Thought, *Why bother?*	"I ate too much tonight and will always overeat and will always be fat."	Overgeneralization	"Okay, I slipped, but I won't give up. I will focus on the here and now. I won't make more of this than there is."

FIGURE 2.1

If you perceive your behavior to be less than perfect, you label yourself a failure. Since you can never reach the incredibly high standards you set for yourself, you will remain locked in a failure loop until you correct your erroneous thinking patterns.

EXERCISE

1. Using the Thought Record, identify each time you engage in all or none thinking this week.

2. What are typical ways you use all or none thinking in relation to food, weight, and body image?

_____

_____

_____

_____

3. What more rational responses can you record?

_____

_____

_____

Overgeneralization

Overgeneralization occurs when a single negative event is seen as a constantly recurring event. With this viewpoint, a single deviation in your weight management efforts may cause you to feel your program has no chance to succeed.

EXERCISE

1. Using the Thought Record, identify and count each time you engage in overgeneralization this week.

WEEK 2

2. Give examples of your overgeneralizing habits regarding weight control, food, and behavior.

_____

_____

_____

_____

3. When you overgeneralize, what feelings follow?

_____

_____

_____

_____

(Note: Additional distorted thinking patterns will be discussed in Thinking sections in ensuing chapters.)

EMOTIONAL:
The Five Levels of
Emotional Healing

Do your feelings fuel your feedings? Last week you learned how your thinking influences your feelings and how negative feelings often precede eating binges. Not all overeating is related to unmet or unresolved emotional needs, but it is worth exploring what connections your past may have with your current weight management struggles. Being unaware of possible root causes may be one reason why weight loss efforts have not worked for you previously.

Studying the following five levels of emotional healing may help you determine if unresolved events in your past are negatively affecting your life:

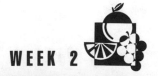

Level 1—Recognize and become aware of real feelings.
Level 2—Label the feelings.
Level 3—Express the feelings.
Level 4—Grieve hurts or losses.
Level 5—Release the past and move on.

The goal of this section is to help you get beyond the hold that past hurts may have on your life. You will explore how childhood experiences may be influencing your current relationship with food. Also, you will learn that repressing such feelings as anger and hurt can create physical and emotional tension, which can result in psychosomatic illness (e.g., high blood pressure, heart disease, gastrointestinal problems).

Psychological tension may be partially relieved by overeating or indulging in some form of addiction; however, resorting to these negative reactions prevents you from seeking and adopting positive solutions. In contrast, when you recognize and appropriately express anger or hurt, enormous tension is released and floodgates of emotion are opened. You experience a sense of peace and well-being as you glimpse the real you. Additionally, as you become more adept at expressing your feelings in an appropriate way as situations arise, you reinforce a greater sense of self. Similar to the transformation in the Christian walk, emotional healing is an ongoing process of change or transformation. The change process we endorse is slow, gentle, and lasting.

In the Christian transformation process, your negative self-concept is replaced by a clear vision of who you are in Christ. You are able to receive the blessings God has promised in His Word. As your knowledge grows and you experience who God is and how precious you are to Him, you lay claim to the power of who you are in Christ. Above all, you experience a closer personal relationship and union with a loving and caring Father who is with you always.

In the emotional healing process, you learn you do not have to remain burdened by hurtful emotional baggage, and you learn how to remove the burdens.

WEEK 2

EXERCISE 1

Review the following, and place a check next to ones you have achieved. Put an "O" next to those you are still working on.

__ 1. Responding to present situations without harmful emotional baggage from the past.

__ 2. Creating healthy relationships based on mutual respect and personal boundaries.

__ 3. Expressing feelings appropriately as situation dictates.

__ 4. Knowing (or learning) how to behave and be treated appropriately.

__ 5. Enjoying the boundless joy and spontaneity within me.

__ 6. Communicating clearly and resolving conflict as it arises.

__ 7. Identifying needs and wishes and taking responsibility for getting them met.

__ 8. Learning where I end and someone else begins.

__ 9. Letting others own and deal with their pain, and not feeling I have to fix them.

__ 10. Feeling I possess a clear self-identity.

__ 11. Feeling I possess strong self-esteem.

__ 12. Not feeling a need to exert control in all situations.

__ 13. Not being controlled.

__ 14. Being able to be more trusting.

__ 15. Giving and receiving love without fear of being hurt and abandoned.

EXERCISE 2

1. In what ways have your changes influenced your food management problem?

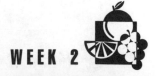

_____

_____

_____

_____

2. In what ways have your changes influenced your relationships with others?

_____

_____

_____

_____

Origins of Pain: Taking Inventory of Your Childhood

This exercise is designed to aid you in understanding your family system, parents or caregivers, siblings, home life, and how each may have influenced you.

Get into a relaxed position. Close your eyes and think back or try to imagine that you are traveling back in time on a train. See yourself when you were in college or of college age. Think back over your high school years. See the friends you had. Try to remember what it was like when you were a teenager. How did you feel about yourself then? What good memories do you recall? What hurts, disappointments, or embarrassments do you remember?

What was your home life like? What was your relationship with your parents or caregivers like when you were a teen? See the train moving back in time before junior high school, back to sixth grade. (Slowly repeat the above questions.)

Now travel back on the train to early elementary school. Can you remember a favorite teacher? A favorite friend? What do you remember wearing? What did you enjoy doing? What do you remember about your birthdays? How were your birthdays celebrated? Did you feel special? Overlooked? What do you remember about holidays? Christ-

WEEK 2

mas? Easter? Birthdays of other family members? What feelings sponta-neously come up when you think back over these events?

Were any relatives alcoholics? Rageaholics? Were holidays fun, re-laxing times? Or wrought with tension, anxiety, and confrontations? Who was usually there? What feelings come up as you remember these events?

Try to imagine the house you lived in when you were young. What rooms do you see? What was your favorite room? What are you doing in that room? Who else is there? Can you see your bedroom? What feelings come up as you reflect on this house? What do you wish could have been different?

Imagine the table where you ate meals. Who do you see sitting there with you? Where did you sit? What does it feel like sitting at that table with those people? What usually went on? How might these mealtime events relate to your current eating habits? What do you wish could have been different?

If you cannot remember all stages described above, you still may see enough for the backward journey to be beneficial. The main focus is to identify as many early influences as possible and determine what role, if any, those influences presently play in your life. Then isolate and learn to let go of any negative emotional baggage such influences engendered.

What Are Basic Needs?

You were born with a need for affection and love, a need to be connected and involved, to be taken care of, and to feel a sense of security and safety. All children need to experience enough attention from their parents or caregivers to feel they are loved and valued. If you are to develop as an emotionally healthy adult, your basic childhood needs must be met. When basic needs are effectively met, you are more likely to have healthy emotional feelings as you mature, and you will be better equipped to offer nurturance to the next generation. A sad

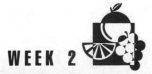

fact is that if your basic needs were not adequately met during child-hood, you may not even know what basic needs are.

Basic needs include the following:

1. Survival and safety (physical needs met)
2. Physical contact (touch, holding, being physically close)
3. Nurturing, love, and unconditional regard
4. Social attention (smiles, verbal affirmations, hugs)
5. Mirroring (communicating or reflecting to the child that needs are understood and needs will be met)
6. Guidance (facilitates learning, provides support while the child shows initiative)
7. Acceptance (feeling of belonging, being valued and admired)
8. Respect (feelings are validated; boundaries are clearly defined; opinions may be expressed freely)
9. Mastery (experience of competence at some things; learning that "I'm good at this")
10. Contentment, joy, and fun (able to relax and enjoy the moment; feeling that now is okay, just as it is)

EXERCISE 1

Review the basic needs listed, and reflect on which needs you feel were not met and at what age. Write down any comments you feel will aid you.

1. Survival and safety: _____

_____

_____.

2. Physical contact: _____

_____

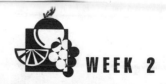

WEEK 2

3. Nurturing, love, and unconditional regard: _____

_____

_____.

4. Social attention: _____

_____

_____.

5. Mirroring: _____

_____

_____.

6. Guidance: _____

_____

_____.

7. Acceptance: _____

_____

_____.

8. Respect: _____

_____

_____.

9. Mastery: _____

_____

_____

_____.

10. Contentment, joy, and fun: _____

_____

_____

_____.

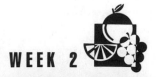

WEEK 2

EXERCISE 2

1. List basic needs you feel were met during your childhood and by whom.

_____
_____
_____
_____
_____

2. Referring to the basic needs that were unmet, can you think of ways to get these needs met now?

_____
_____

3. How have these unmet needs affected your relationships and influenced your problems with food?

_____
_____

EXERCISE 3

1. Review your dietary habits and note whether you gravitate toward food or eating when you feel any of the listed basic needs are not met.

_____
_____
_____

2. Review your answers. Do you detect emotional eating patterns?

_____
_____

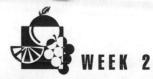

WEEK 2

EXERCISE 4

1. Do you eat a lot of food right before bedtime?

_____

2. What feelings do you experience when you think of the day ending or getting into bed?

_____

3. What are you thinking or feeling while you eat at bedtime?

_____

4. Do you crave food at work because you are bored, stressed out, or insecure?

_____

5. At what other times do you crave food?

_____

6. List several alternative activities you could use as a substitute for food. (Review your logs and journals for alternative activities you have previously listed. Add new ones!)

_____

_____

_____

EXERCISE 5

1. When I was a child, food filled my unmet need(s) for

_____

_____

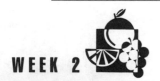

2. When I was a teenager, food filled my unmet need(s) for

_____

_____ .

3. When I was a young adult, food filled my unmet need(s) for

_____

_____ .

4. When I became an adult, food filled my unmet need(s) for

_____

_____ .

PHYSICAL:
Get Ready to Control
Your Weight!

Are you ready to learn healthy weight management? Reviewing the following related areas will help you answer that question.

Motivation

How motivated are you right now to begin your STEP program and gain improved health and permanent weight management? Rate yourself:

__ Not motivated.
__ Somewhat motivated.
__ Very motivated.

Compare your feelings today to any you had previously regarding weight management. How, if at all, do the feelings differ?

Commitment

Losing weight while making significant and lasting lifestyle changes will take commitment through all sections of the STEP program. Each

WEEK 2

is a very important part of the whole. Following these STEPs until they become routine will allow you to continue your program without stress or boredom and you will reap exciting health benefits.

Life Circumstances

Think of the stresses, if any, in your life and how they might interfere with your success. Addressing motivation, commitment, and life circumstances beforehand allows you to smooth your path to success.

To help decide your readiness to make changes, ask yourself the following questions:

1. Does the thought of changing my relationship with food feel overwhelming?

_____

2. Do I feel the need to have everything in order before I make changes in my relationship with food?

_____

3. Can I do it, since I have tried and given up before?

_____

4. If I modify my relationship with food, how will it change my interaction with God?

_____

Family?

_____

Friends?

_____

Some people abandon the program because (1) participation in a diet program becomes too complicated; (2) work, activities, and social events make it too difficult to follow; (3) someone else had the idea for their losing weight; and (4) it is inconvenient, uncomfortable, or upsetting to make choices and stick with them.

Eating healthy food is not difficult, but remaining committed to changes in your lifestyle may present challenges. Answering the following questions may provide insight. Circle yes or no.

YES NO   1. Do I want to change my appearance to please someone else more than for myself?

YES NO   2. Is there a major crisis in my life right now?

YES NO   3. Am I hoping to lose a quick ten to fifteen pounds to look good for an event?

YES NO   4. Is there a payoff for holding on to my weight?

YES NO   5. Will weight loss result in a change in my primary relationships (for example, threaten a spouse)?

YES NO   6. Do I have fears about being thin?

YES NO   7. Will weight loss provide an opportunity to make significant personal changes that I fear (for example, explore other job opportunities, have more visibility)?

YES NO   8. Will losing weight cause me to challenge my current self-concept? Does that scare me?

YES NO   9. Am I facing major changes in my life (for example, a move, marriage, a new baby)?

YES NO   10. Do I have a medical condition that might make weight loss and exercise dangerous?

(A note of caution: A doctor's permission and advice should always be sought if you are pregnant, have high blood pressure, are extremely overweight, or have any other medical condition that should be addressed. It is always best to have a physical checkup before beginning any weight loss or physical exercise program.)

WEEK 2

Analyzing Your Food Buying and Eating Patterns

Answer the following questions to evaluate patterns. Circle yes or no.

YES NO 1. When I crave certain foods to snack on (e.g., cookies, chocolate, chips), do I go to the store?

YES NO 2. Do I go up and down aisles to see what looks good?

YES NO 3. Do I use a shopping list?

YES NO 4. Do I read labels to check grams of sugar, fat, fiber, and protein?

YES NO 5. Am I often hungry when I shop for groceries?

YES NO 6. When I go to the store, do I take index cards with planned recipes specifying ingredients?

YES NO 7. Do I eat while I shop?

EXERCISE

Review your answers; determine and list changes you can make in your shopping behavior to aid your weight control plan.

_____

_____

_____

What Is Healthy Eating?

Healthy eaters are people who generally eat what they want, when they want, without fear of uncontrollable weight gain. They eat to satisfy biological needs instead of emotional ones. Healthy eaters know how to separate physical from emotional hunger cues.

As you progress on your program and continue to adopt new ways of thinking, feeling, and behaving regarding food, healthy eating patterns will develop. (See fig. 2.2.) Good eating behavior must be interwoven with positive views of self-esteem and self-worth. Remember that the Gentle Eating program is a slow, gentle process that develops in small steps and lasts a lifetime.

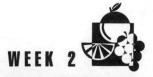

WEEK 2

Generally Recommended Distribution of Daily Calories*

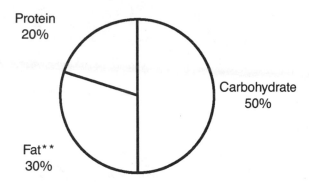

Protein
20%

Carbohydrate
50%

Fat**
30%

*Men, teenagers, and breastfeeding or pregnant women may have different needs.
**Thirty percent, or less, with no more than 10 percent of fat calories from saturated fat.

FIGURE 2.2

Young children are generally healthy eaters who eat to live rather than live to eat. There are usually no body comparisons, obsessive thoughts, fantasies, or guilt about quantity of food or treats consumed. During a typical day, mealtime is only one of many enjoyable events for them wedged between various activities.

Unfortunately, those "various" activities do not include enough physical activity. According to Emily Greenspan Kelting in *Learning to Love Gym,*

> Children today generally are fatter than children were two decades ago, and . . . their cardiovascular fitness lags behind that of active, middle-aged adults. In separate studies in Michigan and Nebraska, 40 percent of the children in elementary school who were tested showed at least one risk factor for developing heart disease—high blood pressure, excessive levels of cholesterol in the blood, obesity, or poor cardiovascular fitness. And last year, less than 4 percent of the 18 million youngsters who took the "President's Challenge"—a test that measures endurance, flexibility, and muscle strength—scored 85 percent or above.

WEEK 2

Apparently, unless otherwise instructed and encouraged, many children prefer skipping physical exercise in favor of sitting mesmerized in front of a television set or playing video games. This provides a handy setting for consuming chips, cookies, candy, and other finger foods high in fat, sodium, and calories. Ongoing studies reveal this behavior is continuing.

Several years ago, the Department of Health and Human Services set forth the following two goals to be achieved by the year 2000: (1) to increase by 30 percent the number of Americans participating in at least a daily half hour of regular, moderate physical activity—from a 1985 level of 22 percent; and (2) to reduce the number of obese Americans by at least 6 percent—from a 1985 level of 26 percent. In a relatively short time those figures will be tallied, and it will be interesting to note whether or not the attempt to educate the public bears fruit. We do not want to be pessimistic, but the past has usually shown that knowing better does not always translate into doing better. However, we have proved to ourselves that when all components of the STEP program are gently and consistently implemented, success is assured.

To keep you and your children from becoming overweight statistics, incorporate Gentle Eating into your family's lifestyle. The results will be healthy souls, healthy minds, and healthy bodies.

Healthy Eating Development Guide

Feel and rate your hunger, using the 0–10 scale (0 = starved, 5 = satisfied, and 10 = stuffed). Think what foods sound good to satisfy that hunger.

Select a moderate portion of foods from all food groups, including beverages.

Select protein, fats, and carbohydrates, including some of the high-calorie foods you may consider forbidden.

Divide your usual three meals equally into six smaller meals. By

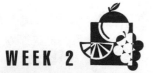

observing the six small meals a day plan, physical hunger is reduced and you are not as likely to overeat.

Eat until you feel full. Wait fifteen to twenty minutes to reevaluate your hunger level, using the 0–10 rating scale: 0 = starved, 5 = satisfied, and 10 = stuffed.

Do not eat less than 1,200 to 1,500 calories a day. After your physical needs are satisfied, it is likely you will think about food less often until another mealtime approaches. Weak hunger feelings come and go, so it is not necessary to react to the first signal.

The Basic Four Daily Nutrition Requirements
(Generally accepted by health professionals)

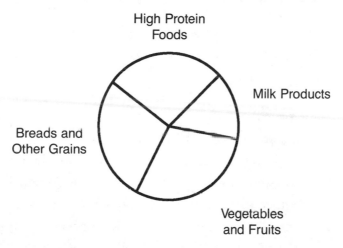

High protein foods (approximately 27.5 percent): two or more servings* daily (meat, seafood, poultry, eggs)

Milk products (approximately 15 percent): one pint to one quart daily**

Vegetables and fruits (approximately 30 percent): four or more servings daily (especially leafy green and yellow vegetables and fresh fruits)

Breads/other grains (approximately 27.5 percent): four or more servings daily (enriched or whole grain)

*A serving is generally considered to be one-half cup.

**One quart (three to four glasses) recommended for children and teenagers; for adults, one pint or its equivalent.

FIGURE 2.3

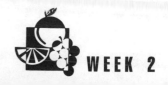

WEEK 2

Meal Plans

Meal plans can be helpful in regulating your habit of overeating (or undereating, which can trigger overeating), and creating healthy varied menus can be enjoyable and rewarding. Consider the following suggestions to develop healthy eating habits:

- Set an eating schedule that suits your needs instead of eating according to usual dietary rules, such as having three large meals per day at set times.
- Have a special table setting and a special place to eat so your meal has a clear beginning and ending, and afterward you can leave the area and food cues behind.
- Most important, *do not skip meals!*

If you still have strong urges to overeat after the first few weeks of Gentle Eating, the following strategies can help you better cope.

1. Use positive statements, such as,

    - "This urge is strong now, but I know it often goes away in a few minutes. Hunger signals come and go and increase over time. I will rate the intensity now and again when it returns."
    - "One reason I want to keep eating, even though I just had an adequate meal, is that my stomach is not yet signaling to me I am full. If I wait fifteen minutes or so, I will probably feel satisfied. There is no need to binge now."
    - "I will trust myself. I am confusing my emotions with my urge to overeat. The urge I feel right now is not a physical one, because I have already eaten enough regular normal meals."
    - "What am I thinking and feeling? What do I need to do to deal with these emotions now, other than eat?"

2. Do not immediately turn to food; continue eating or abstaining in a healthy manner. Focus on helpful coping statements, such as,

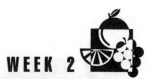

- "This food will not lead to uncontrollable weight gain; I am just nourishing my body."
- "Eating normal meals is a necessary part of feeling better."
- "I know my hunger and full cues are confusing to me now, so I must eat according to my schedule."
- "Smaller meals at regular intervals are more satisfying."
- "I must take in food to nourish my body just like I would give my children medicine and good food."
- "Even if I overeat, slips are okay. I can learn from them and move forward."

3. Generate encouraging remarks to counter the following discouraging ones:

- "I have not lost more than two to five pounds over the last two-week period."
- "I have been skipping exercise because I do not feel like doing it."
- "My progress is going so slow, I feel like quitting."
- "My ideal goal seems too far off."
- "Other people seem to lose weight more easily than I do."
- "Relatives and friends tell me that I do not need to lose any more weight."
- "I lapsed in all categories for four days."
- "After the initial weight loss, I've started to doubt I can continue my program."
- "I feel a surge of fear I will regain all my weight."
- "I fear the loss of positive attention if I regain weight."
- "My spouse puts me down for going off my plan."

4. Break your old dietary rules slowly. If you have a rule that says you can't eat breakfast, try eating a little bit. Leave the eating area at the point when you begin feeling discomfort. Gradually increase the amount you eat and the length of time you stay in the eating area until you eat a healthy meal. This will prevent

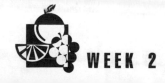

WEEK 2

you from giving up and giving in to the urge to overeat. Eventually, you will leave behind illogical diet rituals that have robbed you of healthy eating and weight control.

5. Gradually introduce foods you have denied yourself, such as bread, chocolate, or pasta. By eating small portions of foods you have been overeating, you can eat them in a responsible, moderate way. Since these foods will no longer be forbidden, you probably will not dwell on them or become anxious and guilty after eating them.

6. Try to eat moderate portions, and let go of diet myths that might have controlled your eating behavior. If you are unsure what a standard portion is, use one cup, one-half cup, and one-fourth cup measuring cups, and you will learn how much satisfies your hunger.

7. If it is difficult for you to digest normal portions, remind yourself that it may be easier for you to eat smaller meals daily rather than three larger meals.

8. Think of ways to involve yourself in other activities once you have finished a meal. Keep a list of activities handy and refer to them often.

9. Pamper yourself. Plan things you enjoy doing each day, even if you have a limited amount of time. When you are well-nourished emotionally, you will be less likely to turn to food.

EXERCISE

1. Can you recall memories of what food meant to you at different ages in your life? What role did food play? What worries or concerns did you have about food?

_____

_____

_____

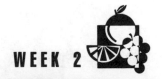

WEEK 2

2. How did the attitudes of your parents or caregivers, siblings, and friends influence your view of food at different ages? If you can recall, jot down your reactions: what you thought, felt, said, and heard about food.

_____

_____

_____

3. What was your family's general attitude regarding food?

_____

_____

_____

4. How did this attitude influence your relationship with food? (For instance, "I should eat everything in front of me"; "If I eat, I will feel better.")

_____

_____

A Gentle "We Told You So": The Ten-Minute Workout

Until recently, most exercise instructors believed and claimed that working out less than twenty consecutive minutes was a waste of time. Anything less than a strenuous, sometimes painful, workout was considered to have little fitness value.

Dr. Kenneth Cooper, president and founder of the Cooper Aerobics Center, Dallas, Texas, in an interview published in _Bottom Line/Personal_ (November 1, 1995), stated,

> During the 30 years I have studied the link between health and fitness, my ideas about how to exercise have changed substantially. In 1968—around the time I invented the term aerobics—I believed a high level of exercise that stimulated the heart was necessary for a long, healthy life. At the time, it appeared that the more you

WEEK 2

exercised, the better off you would be—and unless you were exercising to become aerobically fit, you were wasting your time. Today, medical research shows that you can exercise moderately and gain many of the same benefits.

Findings released in October 1995, regarding studies undertaken at the University of Pittsburgh, revealed that women who were told to exercise in ten-minute bouts four times a day exercised more and lost more weight than women told to exercise for forty minutes once a day. Most of the women chose walking for their exercise, and the ones who exercised in short bouts lost about twenty pounds after twenty-six weeks, while the ones who exercised in longer stretches lost about thirteen pounds.

These findings affirm the Gentle Eating plan for long-term weight management and underscore the value of a stress-free, gentle exercise program. We, the authors of *Gentle Eating*, experienced the effectiveness of adopting a moderate exercise routine, and we know the approach produced lasting results. The Gentle Eating method works and represents a lifestyle change you can enjoy, not a diet plan you must endure. So, set aside a few minutes several times a day for physical activity and tone up and trim down.

Simple Weight Training

Lean muscle has very little fat and burns more calories than under-developed muscle (flab). Keeping your muscles lean requires physical resistance that can be achieved by lifting light weights several minutes daily. If you have your doctor's permission, you can follow this simple, gentle workout.

You need three-, four-, and five-pound hand weights or equivalent weights using water- or sand-filled plastic bottles. A half-gallon container filled with water weighs about four and one-half pounds, and

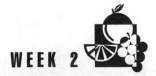

filled with sand, about seven and one-half pounds. Double weight amounts for gallon size. You do not have to fill the containers completely; approximate and determine a comfortable weight.

Easy Exercises for Lifetime Tone Ups

Keeping your arms down at your sides, hold one weight in each hand against each thigh. Slowly lift your arms parallel to the floor or ground. Slowly return your arms to the original position. Repeat gradually five to ten times.

Hold weights next to your thighs (starting position). Bend your arms up, then continue the motion to lift weights over your head. Repeat slowly five to ten times.

Triceps. Hold weights next to your thighs. Slowly raise both forearms so they are parallel to the floor or ground and make a ninety-degree angle. Slowly lower weights to the starting position. Return to the ninety-degree angle and repeat movement five to ten times.

Hold weights with your arms extended downward. Slowly shrug your shoulders (lifting weights with shoulder muscles). Repeat five to ten times.

Legs. Hold weights against thighs. Slowly squat, then rise. (Do not squat to a position that is uncomfortable.) Repeat five to ten times.

Using weights, bend your arms up and hold weights against your chest. Slowly slide one leg forward as far as you comfortably can while keeping the other leg stationary; then return your leg to the starting position. Repeat movement shifting to the other leg. Repeat five to ten times per leg.

Arm Curl. Hold weights, arms extended downward at sides with palms facing forward. Alternately curl weights in each arm upward, keeping elbows at the same level each time. Slowly repeat five to ten times per arm.

Have weights handy and do any combination of these simple exercises at structured or random times. Over time you will notice better

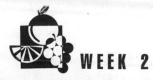

WEEK 2

muscle tone and increased strength. Remember to keep your routines short and simple.

Ankle Weights. Strap a light ankle weight on each leg, and do leg lifts standing or sitting; to the side one at a time while standing, or together when sitting. Slowly repeat movements five to ten times. (Do not overdo.)

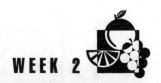

PROGRESS CHART

Check all that apply.

Spiritual Changes

___ Had at least a fifteen-minute daily quiet time.

___ Memorized a Bible verse.

___ Met with midweek church group.

___ Went to church services.

___ Prayed.

___ Felt a little closer to the Lord.

___ Expressed true feelings to God.

___ Honestly evaluated my relationship with God.

Thinking Changes

___ Recognized and recorded a distorted thought.

___ Experienced change in how I view myself.

___ Experienced change in how I thought about a situation.

___ Was able to develop more accurate/balanced view of person, event, etc.

Emotional Changes

___ Recorded my feelings.

___ Evaluated feelings before eating.

___ Expressed feelings in appropriate manner.

___ Noticed impact a person, place, or event had on my urge to eat.

___ Identified a past trauma or hurt.

___ Sought support from a trusted person.

___ Expressed hurt or pain in appropriate way.

___ Noticed how past hurt was related to urge to eat.

___ Worked on a stage of grief.

___ Noticed a change in level of a negative emotion.

___ Noticed a different reaction to person, place, or event that used to evoke emotional upset.

___ Implemented clear, personal emotional boundaries.

 **WEEK 2**

PROGRESS CHART

Check all that apply.

Physical/Behavioral Changes

___ Charted my eating patterns.

___ Did workbook exercises.

___ Tried a new low-fat recipe.

___ Performed at least ten minutes of physical activity.

___ Listened to or watched ten to twenty minutes of a relaxation tape (audio or video).

___ Took at least fifteen minutes for myself.

___ Left some food on my plate.

___ Set a nice table with special touches: flowers, tablecloth, candles; listened to soothing music during mealtime; used special dishes.

___ Went shopping when not hungry.

___ Ate intended portions and stopped.

___ Rated hunger level before and after meals.

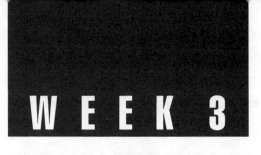

WEEK 3

SPIRITUAL:
Self-Doubt and Fear

■ Moses was so wrought with fear and self-doubt that he didn't want to answer God's call. "But I'm not the person for a job like that!" Moses exclaimed. God answered Moses, saying, "I will certainly be with you" (Ex. 3:11–12 TLB).

The personal changes you need to make may seem monumental, perhaps impossible. However, great biblical leaders had character flaws, shortcomings, and struggles similar to yours, and God molded them and was able to use them for great works. Are you willing to let God mold and change you for future work He has for you?

At times your fear of change may be greater than your faith. Making changes and giving up your reliance on food as a comfort and method of contending with difficulties require faith in God's promises to help you in your times of need.

Genesis 12:10–20 relates that as Abram was approaching Egypt's border, he became gripped with fear that he would be killed and the Egyptians would take his wife, Sarai. Instead of trusting God, Abram took matters into his hands and said that Sarai was his sister. Genesis 26:1–11 reveals how Abram's son, Isaac, became fearful and concocted a similar story to protect his life. Although Abram and Isaac should have put their trust in God to protect them, fear ruled their thoughts.

WEEK 3

In both instances, there would have been tragic consequences if not for the Lord's intervention.

EXERCISE 1

1. Do you trust God for small things but panic when faced with larger issues?

_____

2. Are there times when you turn to food instead of God to calm your fears?

_____

If you answered yes, give examples of the times.

_____
_____
_____

You can trust in these words:

> You shall eat in plenty and be satisfied,
> And praise the name of the LORD your God,
> Who has dealt wondrously with you;
> And My people shall never be put to shame (Joel 2:26).
>
> For the Lord GOD will help Me;
> Therefore I will not be disgraced;
> Therefore I have set My face like a flint,
> And I know that I will not be ashamed (Isa. 50:7).

EXERCISE 2

1. Do you consider yourself "bad" or your behavior "undesirable"? Write some examples here.

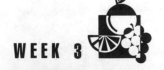

_____

_____

_____

2. In what ways, if any, do you experience shame with regard to your food issues?

_____

_____

_____

Turning Negative into Positive

Though you may feel victimized by circumstances that were beyond your control (e.g., you were too young to seek help or even perhaps to know that help might be available), you do not have to adopt a lifetime label of victim. Only in facing the realities of your situation can you recover from problems you might have inherited. Read God's Word and learn that when you stay knitted closely to God and focus on God's will for your life, you will reap the blessings of God's infinite power and protection. If you remain steadfast in your devotion to God and have faith and courage, God will deliver you from difficult circumstances.

EXERCISE

1. How can you give more of yourself to God?

_____

_____

2. What changes would take place in your life by following God's will and not your own?

_____

_____

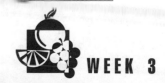 **WEEK 3**

3. When the outcome of God's call is not clear, do you compromise? How?

_____

_____

Heeding God's Call

Moses, Job, and many other leaders in the Bible did not always fully understand the commands God gave them. Nevertheless, they did what God asked, and in the end they were victorious. The positive outcome of God's call may not be immediately obvious, but focus on your ultimate reward: eternal life with the Lord, your Father.

"Let Go and Let God"

Perhaps you were born into a family that had a negative impact on your life and you endured a painful childhood. The good news is this: The story does not have to end there. As you learned earlier, you can face your pain and the problems it caused and leave it behind. Read the story of Daniel; he has many lessons to teach you.

Daniel and his friends were innocent bystanders who were exiled to Babylon because of Judah's prolonged disobedience to God. But Daniel didn't use the punishment he inherited as an excuse to give up. Daniel stood firm in his faith despite repeated suffering, and he refused to compromise his values and beliefs. He set clear boundaries for his behavior, and he stood by those decisions against seemingly overwhelming odds. Because of Daniel's faith and courage, God not only repeatedly delivered him from harsh situations but also used Daniel to prove His existence and power to others. Daniel was more than a survivor; he was an overcomer. Heed these words:

> That Christ may dwell in your hearts through faith; that you, being rooted and grounded in love, may be able to comprehend with all the saints what is the width and length and depth and height—to know

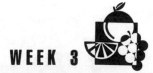

WEEK 3

the love of Christ which passes knowledge; that you may be filled with all the fullness of God (Eph. 3:17–19).

EXERCISE

1. Does your faith sometimes weaken? Think of ways to build and strengthen your faith.

_____

_____

2. What important lessons can you learn from Daniel?

_____

_____

3. Because of Daniel's steadfast faith and courage, God delivered Daniel. Can you think of an instance when God was able to use you in this way?

_____

_____

Feeling Left Out, Worthless, and Alone

Read the story of Hagar and Ishmael (Gen. 21). They experienced rejection and alienation from their community. Think how helpless and hopeless Hagar and her son must have felt. They were cast aside by those who had once esteemed them. You can learn from the plight of Hagar and Ishmael how God can help you build a strong sense of self-worth and self-esteem despite present realities.

To receive God's blessings and help, put your faith in His promises, and call on Him to be Lord over your life. God's love for you and His concern for your welfare are enduring and unfailing. Jesus said, "If you abide in Me, and My words abide in you, you will ask what you desire, and it shall be done for you" (John 15:7).

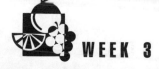

WEEK 3

EXERCISE

1. Have you called on God to be Lord over your life?

_____

2. Recall Hagar's story. How does it minister to you?

_____

_____

_____

3. If you have not called on God, can you think what might be blocking your way?

_____

_____

_____

4. Do you feel you have experienced rejection and alienation because of a weight problem? Do you have these feelings at home, in public, at your place of employment?

_____

_____

_____

5. Seek God's help and His shield against harsh treatment directed toward you. Note some changes that will allow you to have a more positive self-image.

_____

_____

_____

God's Power Will Prevail

Addictions will always fail you as a means for coping with pain and life's challenges. Consuming large amounts of food or drugs or turning

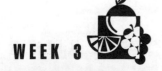

to destructive behavior will never solve your problems. Such behavior will increase them. Attempting to rely on your own resources and doing the best you know how to do is a good second step. However, the first, most important, and most powerful one is always calling on God. Don't waste another minute thinking you can or must handle your problems alone. God is with you; turn to Him in prayer.

Jeremiah 10:4–5 reminds us that trusting in addictions as a substitution for God's power is like raising up an idol. It is wrong and can have no good or positive results. Think of the awesome power God possesses! He will help you overcome your addictions.

You need strong spiritual faith and guidance, and God is the source. He will aid you; help is only a prayer away. You can begin by praying, "Lord, I am discouraged and weary from my lonely struggles. I want and need Your help." Continue to talk with Him as your heart dictates. Peace will permeate your life as you feel His power, and His power will prevail.

EXERCISE

1. Read Ezekiel 23:1–49 and 2 Thessalonians 1:3–5. Can you see a relationship between these passages and dependency on food instead of seeking God's help?

_____

2. Read 2 Corinthians 3. Does that Scripture help you realize God's power allows you to make changes in your life? Note how it emphasizes change is possible!

_____

_____

3. Record ways that God's power can change you from within.

_____

_____

WEEK 3

4. Remember that all success comes from God. Seek out Scriptures that reaffirm and strengthen your faith; cite the references here as reminders.

_____

_____

_____

Lord, my days and nights have been filled with joy since I gave my life into Your keeping. I now know that You were always there, waiting patiently for me to turn to You for strength and guidance. I had tried unsuccessfully to manage my problems and obsessive eating habits, thinking that I could change them without help. I felt like a failure, and unhealthy thoughts clouded my mind. I thank You for replacing my negative thoughts with positive hopes. The peace and comfort I have found in You have allowed me to make a new beginning, with my spirit revived and hopes renewed. With You in my heart and at my side, I know all things are possible. Amen.

THINKING:
Mental Filter and
Selective Abstraction

You focus on a single negative detail and filter out the positive. You see only the negative with this form of distorted thinking, and your memory bank registers or deposits only negative events and responses. All prior successes lose meaning, and positive gains go unnoticed or do not get processed. Any mistake is selectively used as a focal point indicating total failure.

Did you read the preceding paragraph and automatically think, _That certainly does not apply to me_? When you fill out and review your Thought Record, you may find this thinking pattern is pervasive. No doubt you will be surprised at how often those around you engage in such negative behavior as you listen more closely to their conversations. Some view this behavior as merely a bad habit; in fact, it is highly self-destructive.

As you progress through this workbook, the need to be more thoughtful and gentle in your thinking will become magnified, and you will learn to respond positively to that need.

EXERCISE

1. Record in the Thought Record occurrences of mental filter or selective abstraction.

2. Give examples of how you use mental filter or selective abstraction regarding food, weight control, and behavior.

_____

_____

_____

_____

Emotional Reasoning

You experience negative emotions and conclude those emotions reflect the true state of things. This error in thinking is especially misleading because your feelings follow your thoughts and beliefs. Therefore, if distorted thoughts and beliefs form the basis of your feelings, distorted feelings can be the only outcome.

Because things feel a certain way, you believe they are that way: "I feel like a failure; therefore, I must be a failure." You assume your negative emotions accurately reflect the way things are: "That's the way I feel, so it must be true"; "I feel I'm going to overeat; therefore, I have no control over my behavior." The fact is, you do have power over your thoughts and behavior. Even in the middle of overeating, you can stop and move on to another activity.

WEEK 3

EXERCISE

1. Use the Thought Record to identify and record instances of emotional reasoning.

2. How does emotional reasoning interfere with your weight loss efforts?

_____

_____

_____

EMOTIONAL:
Understanding Your Core Issues

You can learn to identify certain behaviors or character traits that have robbed you of satisfying relationships and real joy in life. Perhaps some areas of your social, emotional, and psychological development were stunted because of a troubled life. If so, your goal of experiencing a happy, healthy life may have been compromised. However, if you adopt positive changes slowly and steadily, you will stay on a direct path to the happy, healthy lifestyle you seek. A step to change and emotional wholeness is identifying and understanding your core issues. (Remember the importance of always treating yourself gently.)

EXERCISE

Check any of the following that might be core issues for you:

___ Need to control (e.g., others, the future, the outcome)

___ Fear of abandonment (being left alone, unloved)

___ Perfectionism (nothing is ever quite good enough)

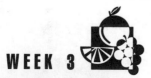

— Codependent (needs/feelings of others are more important than yours)

— Boundary confusion (where you "begin" and "end")

— Low self-esteem ("I'm not worth much")

— Fear of intimacy (difficulty connecting, giving and/or receiving love)

— Difficulty expressing true feelings (for fear of rejection)

— Overly passive (afraid to speak up and assert yourself)

— Overly aggressive (you have to take what's yours)

— Hidden resentment (holding on to past hurts)

— Unresolved grief (denying the pain and hurt of a loss)

— General fearfulness (something bad might happen)

— Self-hatred ("I'm disgusting")

— Difficulty trusting ("I might get hurt")

— Communication problems (especially difficulty with task-oriented, direct problem solving)

— Problem with anger or rage (frequent emotional outbursts)

Parents or caregivers can unknowingly hurt you in ways that have long-term negative effects. Identifying past hurts is not meant to blame your parents or caregivers, who in most instances did the best they knew to do and were probably unaware of any wrongdoing. But understanding how your past may influence your current behaviors and beliefs is necessary to halt self-defeating patterns. There is an emotional pattern to eating, and you can change that pattern.

Defense Mechanisms

From the time you are born, you develop and rely on defense mechanisms in reaction to emotional pain and as a means of coping with daily life. Pushing an incident out of conscious awareness is a common defense mechanism you might have used to endure a difficult emotional experience. However, continued overreliance on defense mechanisms compromises social and emotional growth. You need to deal directly with past emotional issues, including any from childhood,

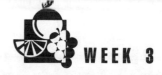

WEEK 3

to promote healthy emotional and personal growth. This is an essential task. As you continue to make gradual, steady gains in your quest for resolutions to your problems, you will be rewarded with a more joyful, less-stressful life.

EXERCISE 1

Check the defense mechanisms you think you rely on most. Note when and how they are triggered.

___ Intellectualization: You stay in your head. You deal with pain in an emotionally detached way.

___

___ Repression: You push painful memories or impulses out of conscious awareness.

___

___ Denial: You behave as though the event never existed or is not occurring.

___

___ Regression: You act or feel as you did at an earlier age (usually as a child).

___

___ Projection: Not wanting to own your undesirable traits or behavior, you assign them to someone else. It's a form of rationalization.

___

___ Hypochondriasis: You have many physical complaints with no apparent physical reasons.

___

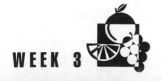

__ Narcissism: You tend to be self-absorbed and egocentric. Only your needs are important. You react with anger to "undeserved" criticism.

__ Reaction formation: You conceal your true motive by giving the opposite, more acceptable one.

__ Passive-aggressive behavior: Unable to assert yourself directly, you exert control or express anger in an indirect, safe way (e.g., showing up late, "accidentally" forgetting, "accidentally" breaking a favorite object).

__ Rationalization: You give logical or socially acceptable motives for your behavior. You make "acceptable" excuses.

Other maladaptive ways of coping may be related to your eating behavior. Check applicable ones, and note when and how they are triggered.

__ Workaholism: Your personal worth is what you achieve; keeping busy keeps you from feeling (or remembering).

__ Sex addiction: Constant preoccupation with sexual material and behavior distracts you from stress or other psychic pain.

__ Alcoholism: Your use of alcohol numbs present or past feelings, emotions, and events.

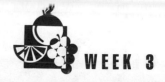

WEEK 3

—— Drug addiction: Your use of drugs numbs present or past feelings, emotions, and events.

———

—— Codependency: You focus primarily on the needs of others at the expense of your own needs. You deny that your needs are important.

———

Although these coping styles help you survive at the time, you ultimately pay a high emotional price. You never realize your full potential, and you never experience a deep sense of love, acceptance, and security. By relying on these coping styles, you are limiting your personal growth and your relationships with others.

1. Review the list of defense mechanisms.

2. From what core issues are these defenses protecting you?

———
———

3. How has the use of these defenses stunted your personal growth?

———
———

4. Review the list of defenses and note the ones you most rely on. Do you feel challenged to adopt more positive coping methods?

———
———

EXERCISE 2

1. How has the use of defense mechanisms limited you emotionally and socially?

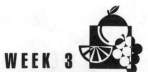

_____

_____

2. Which ones are you ready to give up?

_____

_____

3. List more adaptive ways you can get your needs met.

_____

_____

4. How will you learn to do this?

_____

_____

5. What defenses relate to your problem with food? How?

_____

_____

Knowing Your Real Self

When a child lives in an unhealthy family system, her true self (i.e., who she really is) often is not allowed expression. Over time, she loses connection with her true feelings and develops a false self. The child learns to view reality and to feel and behave in accordance with what the "system" expects and to take the path of least resistance. Perhaps you can identify with this. To survive, you may have had to repress or deny parts of your real self.

Irene was a member of our Gentle Eating group who felt she was not allowed to express her real self. Irene was an only child, and her mother could not have other children. Unfortunately for Irene, her father always wanted a son. At a young age and after much derision by her father, Irene learned to deny, split off, and disown her feminine

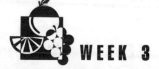

WEEK 3

side. Because her father made fun of her, Irene gave up playing with dolls, dressing up, and wearing dresses. Irene learned that to please Dad, she had to suppress her true self and take on a false self. Although she would rather have worn dresses and played with dolls, she stopped doing both in order to get Dad's approval.

EXERCISE

1. What parts of your true self did you disown or lose during childhood? (For instance, due to a chaotic or unpredictable family environment, you were not able to relax and enjoy carefree playtime. As an adult, you have a difficult time relaxing and having fun.)

_____

_____

_____

2. What experiences in your childhood led to your developing a false self?

_____

_____

_____

The "Good Enough" Parents or Caregivers

Most parents or caregivers were at least adequate in meeting their children's needs. Labeling entire families as either functional or dysfunctional is too general because almost all families function to some extent. Perhaps it is more helpful to think about parenting in terms of a continuum of adequacy in meeting children's needs. At one end of the spectrum is inadequate or unhealthy parenting; at the other end is ideal parenting. In the middle is good enough parenting. Think about your family or the parenting you received. What about it was ideal, good enough, or unhealthy?

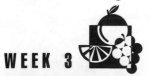

EXERCISE 1

Using the scale, indicate how you would rate the quality of the parenting you received.

Parenting Continuum

Ideal   Good Enough   Inadequate/Unhealthy ·

■——————————————●——————————————■

EXERCISE 2

1. List positive qualities you think you learned or inherited from your parents or caregivers (e.g., a good sense of humor, persistence, honesty, compassion, loyalty).

_____

_____

_____

2. List negative qualities you believe you possess, without regard to origins, that you can work toward changing.

_____

_____

_____

3. How can you begin to gradually and steadily shed negative qualities and focus on adopting positive qualities that will enhance your life?

_____

_____

_____

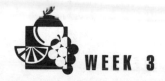 **WEEK 3**

Your Family Role

What was your role in your family of origin? Some roles you were put into as a child might have compromised your emotional and social development. Perhaps both parents worked, and you acted as caregiver during certain hours.

During a Gentle Eating group meeting, Jason shared information about his family role. When Jason was ten years old, he was responsible for preparing breakfast for himself and his five-year-old sister, walking her to and from school each day, preparing their dinner, and caring for her until his mother returned home from work at 6:30 P.M. The pattern continued for many years.

As an adult, Jason remembered his earlier years and recalled repressing his fears of being in charge of his younger sister as well as taking care of his own needs and often being without parental guidance. He became a perfectionist, an overachiever, and an overeater. The "overdoing" in his career might have helped him cope with his deep inner fear of being vulnerable at such a young age. Perhaps the excessive behaviors also gave him a sense of control over his world. He reported that at the age of ten, he felt helpless when adult problems arose. He was often unable to figure out what to do, yet he had to appear in control. Former latchkey kids report similar feelings.

Marsha, another Gentle Eating group member, shared her story. Marsha's parents had a very unhappy marriage. By the time Marsha was seven, her mother used her as a confidante, and Marsha heard daily about all the things her father did wrong and the pain that he caused her mother. Marsha felt that she couldn't say anything positive about her father in her mother's presence. She felt guilty and confused when she expressed love toward her father. She was put into the role of her mother's team member, having to sit and listen daily to negative comments about her father. Marsha realized that she had often looked for something to eat during and after her mother's tirades. Somehow, food helped her deal with the upset. As an adult, she turned to food when she felt unsure or guilty in her relationships.

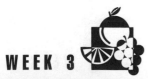

Try to recall the roles you were forced into while you were growing up. Do these roles influence how you deal with life today? In the exercise below, evaluate the roles you were unfairly (and, probably, unintentionally) pushed into as a child. Next, try to determine how your early roles influenced your current behavior.

EXERCISE 1

What were your nicknames?

_____

How did you feel when you were addressed by such names?

_____

_____

What role did such nicknames limit you to?

_____

_____

How did your family members see you?

_____

_____

_____

What type of person would they say you were?

_____

_____

_____

How do they view you now?

_____

_____

_____

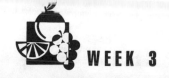

WEEK 3

How is their current view of you similar to their view of you as a child?

_____

_____

How does their current view of you limit your self-expression and potential?

_____

_____

How can you communicate to them the person you are now and the way their distorted, old view of you is limiting current relationships?

_____

_____

Are you ready to set boundaries with them?

_____

_____

What is it like in your home now?

_____

_____

What do you feel like when you first get home?

_____

_____

After a stressful day, do you eat to relax?

_____

What other alternatives to eating can you think of?

_____

_____

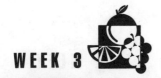

WEEK 3

What is it like as you prepare or wait for meals?

_____

_____

_____

What does it feel like sitting at your table during meals now?

_____

_____

_____

In what ways do your mealtimes or feelings influence your eating behavior?

_____

_____

_____

EXERCISE 2

Consider the roles listed below. If you were put into any of these roles, note how it influenced your current behavior and your relationship with food.

Mother (to whom)?

_____

_____

Father (to whom)?

_____

_____

Parent's or caregiver's confidant(e)?

_____

_____

WEEK 3

Peacemaker (for parents or caregivers)?

_____

_____

Peacemaker (for quarreling siblings)?

_____

_____

Caregiver (for whom)?

_____

_____

The "good at everything" child (to satisfy parent's or caregiver's ego)?

_____

_____

The scapegoat (things were always your fault; bad things happened because of you)?

_____

_____

The assertive or brave one (because parents or caregivers were not)?

_____

_____

The joker (to ease family tensions, keep family members "happy")?

_____

_____

Other role(s)?

_____

_____

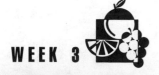

WEEK 3

Gauging Emotional Closeness

In enmeshed families, it is difficult to tell where personal boundaries of family members begin and end. Respect for the needs and rights of family members is lacking. Aid in the fulfillment of the needs of family members is seldom, if ever, offered. In codependent relationships, another person's needs become one's own. One's needs are deemed less important than the needs of the other person. Healthy relationships, by contrast, acknowledge the needs and rights of others and are respectful of boundaries. Individuality is encouraged. Members are supported and esteemed. Closeness is possible and desired, but so is separateness. Privacy is respected.

In enmeshed families, everyone's personal life is open to invasion and discussion. Differing opinions are not solicited and are often punished (e.g., saying, "What a stupid idea!").

Distant or disconnected families are like uninvolved roommates. They live under the same roof but show very little emotional connection. Not involved in each other's business, they behave as if they do not care. In distant families, little personal closeness and warmth are shown; few personal feelings are expressed. Similar to the enmeshed family, there is very little encouragement for individual growth.

By contrast, healthy families have an ongoing relaxing and contracting of closeness, depending on the situation. When feelings, opinions, and boundaries are respected, children learn to trust and respect themselves and others. They feel comfortable taking risks, and they are able to assert themselves when their boundaries have been violated.

EXERCISE

Recall the emotional closeness you experienced in your family of origin. Perhaps your family has characteristics of both extremes on the emotional closeness scale. Using the following scale, put an X at the point that would best describe your family.

93

WEEK 3

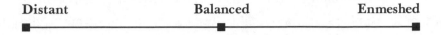

Emotional Closeness Continuum

Distant	Balanced	Enmeshed

Now, think back about individual family members and how they could be rated (for instance, you/Mom, Tom/Dad, Jane/you, etc.). You might gain insight by showing the ratings, using the above format. Create as many scales as you choose.

How did the type of family you grew up in influence your relationship with food? (One Gentle Eating group member stated that there was so much verbal fighting going on at the table, her stomach was in knots at almost every meal. She wouldn't eat then, but she would overeat later while alone in her bedroom.)

_____

_____

_____

Taking a Look at Family Boundaries

Boundaries are barriers that have a beginning and an end, and boundaries in a family are used to define where one person begins and ends or one role begins and ends. Ideally, the family system has clear boundaries. Parents or caregivers come first and are responsible for the children's physical, spiritual, and emotional welfare. Parents or caregivers are responsible for handling financial matters, planning meals, and providing for the children's needs. Parents' or caregivers' emotional and psychological needs are primarily met by each other or other adults; these needs include companionship, romance, and affirmation.

Ideally, parents or caregivers resolve their conflicts with clear communication, negotiation, and compromise, if necessary. Children are not brought into the middle of parental or adult conflicts. The levels of authority are clearly delineated and communicated through reasonable discipline. Children are expected to perform roles in keeping with their

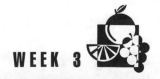

emotional and physical development. In a healthy family, there is respect for each family member's person, belongings, feelings, strengths, and challenges.

EXERCISE

1. Were your boundaries respected as a child or teen?

_____

2. If you answered no, in what way(s) were your boundaries invaded?

_____

_____

_____

3. By whom?

_____

_____

4. Do you see any relationship with your family boundaries and your ability to keep healthy boundaries with food? (For example, do your meals have a beginning and an end?)

_____

_____

_____

PHYSICAL:
Identify Trigger Events

Review your food diary. Can you identify people, activities, and surroundings that make you crave certain foods? For example, if you have a presentation at work, do you turn to food to calm you or to

WEEK 3

soothe anxieties about your performance? If a friend or your spouse puts you down, do you turn to food for comfort? If your feelings are hurt because you are not invited to a social event that many of your friends are attending, do you turn to food? If you make a mistake at work, do you eat to feel better? You're alone at home, and your spouse is late again; would a fudge brownie and ice cream make things better?

EXERCISE 1

1. List your trigger events. These will become more obvious as you continue your food diary.

People: _____

_____.

Activities: _____

_____.

Situations: _____

_____.

Emotions: _____

_____.

2. What do you need to learn to do instead?

_____

_____

EXERCISE 2

1. What did you need from parents or caregivers but did not get?

_____

_____

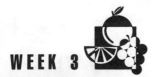

2. What do you wish parents or caregivers could have done differently to make you feel more loved, more accepted, special and worth spending time with, and more secure?

_____

_____

3. How do these unmet needs relate to your problems with food?

_____

_____

Amount of Physical Activity

You may initially resist planning time for exercise when you begin your weight management program. Nevertheless, moderate physical activity performed daily is necessary to long-term weight control, and a gentle daily exercise program is a good starting point. You may choose to increase your daily physical activity, but keep the exercises short and moderate. Studies show average dieters soon abandon weight loss and exercise programs, perhaps because of burnout or boredom.

By following the Gentle Eating plan and keeping your long-term goals in mind, you will succeed in managing your weight. You will begin to view physical activity as an enjoyable method of staying healthy and fit and not approach it with dread. One thing is clear: If lifetime weight control is your goal, you must move, move, and keep moving!

EXERCISE

1. When you think of exercise, what comes to mind?

_____

2. How do these thoughts or expectations influence your desire to exercise?

_____

3. To successfully control your weight, do you need to adopt a different view?

_____

_____

4. How can you transform a new view into gentle, positive physical action?

_____

_____

Put On Your Creative Thinking Cap

Many people, especially parents of young children, often say that exercise is a luxury; there is no way they can do one more thing. But if you are flexible and creative, you can think of activities that keep you moving more each day, increasing your weight loss and overall fitness.

EXERCISE

1. List ideas for moderately increasing your daily physical activity.

_____

_____

2. For activities listed that you are willing to try, indicate when you will try them. Scheduling a time will aid you in getting started.

- Take preschooler in stroller for brisk fifteen- to twenty-minute walk.
  (When? _____)
- Walk to park and walk or jog while I watch kids play.
  (When? _____)
- Briskly walk up and down stairs instead of walking slowly. (Use caution!)
  (When? _____)

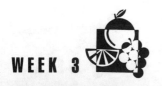

WEEK 3

- Park car a little farther away from store entrances.
  (When? _____)
- Find an indoor place to walk or jog during bad weather.
  (When? _____)
- Begin my walk or jog even when I don't feel like it. After a minute or so notice how I feel and whether I want to continue. (Discontinue immediately if in pain or distress.)
  (When? _____)
- Do light bending and stretching exercises for two to three minutes.
  (When? _____)
- Walk or jog behind a child riding a bike or tricycle.
  (When? _____)
- Move briskly during housecleaning activities.
  (When? _____)
- If possible, swim ten to fifteen minutes two to three times weekly.
  (When? _____)
- If at work, walk during lunch hour and eat lunch at desk (slowly).
  (When? _____)

Keep long-term goals in focus. Slowly and gently is a workable method of exercising.

Poll results indicate four-fifths of Americans do not exercise regularly. Perhaps the thought of exercising every day overwhelms them, so they do nothing. The Gentle Eating program is one you can live with!

"Eat Everything on Your Plate or Someone Might Starve"

Were you taught, or forced, to eat everything on your plate? Many parents or caregivers were taught that eating everything on the plate ensured healthier kids, and they continued the practice with their children. Some might have been taught waste was a sin. Somehow kids in

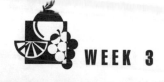

WEEK 3

other parts of the world suffered if you wasted food, and for their sake you ate it. The tactic was, no doubt, employed with the best intentions to make you grateful you had food when many were deprived.

Though such thinking is totally illogical, it became an effective ploy to make children eat every morsel on their plates. This is not a healthy method of dealing with food consumption. Take care not to use this method with your children because it may become a basis for problems with weight management.

EXERCISE 1

1. How do you feel when you leave food on your plate?

_____

2. When you were growing up, what message did you receive if you did not eat all your food?

_____

_____

3. Who usually dished up your portions?

_____

4. Thinking back, how did you feel when someone served you food?

_____

_____

5. What foods did you dislike that you were forced to eat?

_____

6. How did you feel forcing them down?

_____

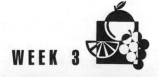

7. What message did you receive about trusting your internal hunger cues?

_____

_____

Being forced or coerced to eat food against your will might have contributed to the development of an eating disorder. If your stomach's signal of fullness or dislike for a particular food was ignored by your parents or caregivers, you might have lost your ability to correctly read your signals.

Some parents or caregivers, teachers, and other adults praise kids who eat a variety of foods as being good eaters. Picky or finicky eaters are often seen in a less-desirable light. Many parents believe picky eaters will be "cured" if they are forced to eat many different foods. Again, the stomach's signal of hunger or like or dislike of a particular food is invalidated, and the picky eater might feel punished for reading food signals accurately.

EXERCISE 2

1. Were you considered a good eater? ____ By whom?

_____

2. Were you considered a picky eater? ____ By whom?

_____

3. What positive or negative attention did you receive because of your eating style?

_____

_____

From whom?

_____

Sandy garnered attention for eating a lot. A middle child in a family of six children, she took attention any way she could get it. At mealtime she forced herself to eat multiple helpings. She wanted to stand out among her five brothers and sisters as being the best eater, especially pleasing Mom, who was the cook. Unfortunately, Sandy ignored her signal of fullness and ignored her body's indication of not liking particular foods. She gradually lost the ability to know when she was hungry or full and what foods she liked and disliked.

EXERCISE 3

1. What food-related attention (positive or negative) or punishment did you receive as a child?

_____

_____

2. How has this influenced your current relationship with food?

_____

_____

3. Are you ready to give up these old, irrational beliefs?

_____

If not, explore why you cling to such beliefs.

_____

_____

_____

4. What messages will you pack up and leave behind?

_____

_____

_____

5. What freedom will this allow you?

_____

_____

6. What more constructive thought or behavior change will you substitute to get this need for attention met?

_____

_____

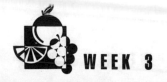 **WEEK 3**

PROGRESS CHART

Check all that apply.

Spiritual Changes

___ Had at least a fifteen-minute daily quiet time.

___ Memorized a Bible verse.

___ Met with midweek church group.

___ Went to church services.

___ Prayed.

___ Felt a little closer to the Lord.

___ Expressed true feelings to God.

___ Honestly evaluated my relationship with God.

Thinking Changes

___ Recognized and recorded a distorted thought.

___ Experienced change in how I view myself.

___ Experienced change in how I thought about a situation.

___ Was able to develop more accurate/balanced view of person, event, etc.

Emotional Changes

___ Recorded my feelings.

___ Evaluated feelings before eating.

___ Expressed feelings in appropriate manner.

___ Noticed impact a person, place, or event had on my urge to eat.

___ Identified a past trauma or hurt.

___ Sought support from a trusted person.

___ Expressed hurt or pain in appropriate way.

___ Noticed how past hurt was related to urge to eat.

___ Worked on a stage of grief.

___ Noticed a change in level of a negative emotion.

___ Noticed a different reaction to person, place, or event that used to evoke emotional upset.

___ Implemented clear, personal emotional boundaries.

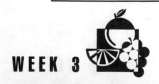

WEEK 3

104

PROGRESS CHART

Check all that apply.

Physical/Behavioral Changes

___ Charted my eating patterns.

___ Did workbook exercises.

___ Tried a new low-fat recipe.

___ Performed at least ten minutes of physical activity.

___ Listened to or watched ten to twenty minutes of a relaxation tape (audio or video).

___ Took at least fifteen minutes for myself.

___ Left some food on my plate.

___ Set a nice table with special touches: flowers, tablecloth, candles; listened to soothing music during mealtime; used special dishes.

___ Went shopping when not hungry.

___ Ate intended portions and stopped.

___ Rated hunger level before and after meals.

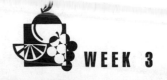

WEEK 3

SPIRITUAL:
Boundaries

■ Exodus 18:13–26 tells about the difficulty Moses had in setting boundaries with his people. "You're going to wear yourself out trying to do it all," Jethro warned. At times Moses pushed himself beyond any limit God expected of him.

Set appropriate personal boundaries with family, friends, coworkers, and acquaintances. When you try to be all things to all people, without realizing it you may be trying to play God, and your life will become out of balance. Allowing others to take advantage of you is detrimental to you and your relationships with others.

When demands on your time overwhelm you, you need to reserve personal time and space to walk and talk with God and set priorities. Try to do this in a gentle manner, but stand firm in your commitment to set aside time to reflect, renew, and recharge.

In Genesis, God's Word tells you that He created you in His image. He made the land, seas, sun, moon, animals, and all things, but only people did He make in His image. Then God breathed life into people. What a unique, close, and intimate relationship you have with God!

> Blessed be Your glorious name,
> Which is exalted above all blessing and praise!
> You alone are the LORD;

WEEK 4

You have made heaven,
The heaven of heavens, with all their host,
The earth and everything on it,
The seas and all that is in them,
And You preserve them all.
The host of heaven worships You (Neh. 9:5–6).

EXERCISE

1. Does the fact God created you in His image change your view of yourself?

_____

2. Does this fact change your view of others?

_____

3. Have you used the excuse, "God loves me unconditionally, no matter how I look or how much I weigh or how upset or moody I become"?

_____

4. If you have used the above excuse to avoid losing weight or controlling your emotions, you are making God's unconditional love a weakness in your life rather than a powerful strength. God wants you to realize your full potential in life, and that includes looking your best, feeling your best, and acting your best! Describe ways to leave excuses behind.

_____
_____
_____

Learning to Deal with People Who Pull You Down

Are there family members or others who hurt you with verbal and emotional abuse? Setting personal boundaries will aid you in removing

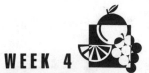

yourself from such harmful treatment. It is not enough to feel some of them may not be aware of the consequences of their actions or the destruction they cause. By God's commandment, you are required to love them, but you are not required to be hurt and suffer in the process.

Many Christians were brought up in family environments where certain emotions were not allowed to be expressed. Christians sometimes feel the expression of anger is not biblical. In many instances, turning the other cheek is taken to the extreme, allowing others to invade personal boundaries. While trying to be good Christians, many people have been verbally abused, and they have permitted others to take advantage of them by not asserting themselves. In the process, emotions were repressed, and food was often used to abate anger and frustration.

You do not help fellow Christians grow to spiritual maturity if you allow them to invade your boundaries. Respectful, clear, assertive communication is not only Christian; it is scriptural.

These invisible boundaries you are building will act as walls or barriers protecting you from abuse or misuse by others. Learn to construct healthy boundaries regarding what you will and will not permit others to say or do to you. Do this as gently as possible, but do not swerve from your goal.

Also, set boundaries to keep your destructive behaviors in check. Making sure trigger foods are not readily available is one healthy boundary against your eating wrong foods. Spending more time with God and seeking out friends who are trying to improve their quality of life will stem temptations you might otherwise encounter.

EXERCISE

1. Think of situations where setting personal boundaries would help you in your relationships with others. List them.

_____

_____

WEEK 4

2. What personal boundaries could you set that would aid you in developing healthier eating habits?

_____

_____

3. List some new relationships you might seek that would enhance your life.

_____

_____

_____

4. List some instances when you turned the other cheek and later felt you should have been more assertive.

_____

_____

_____

5. What feelings did you repress while you were growing up? Name them and write down the effect of such repression on your life.

_____

_____

Do You Refuse to Stop Till You Drop?

Do you overeat in response to feeling excessively tired? When you are faced with deadlines at home or work, the daily stress of life can sometimes seem overwhelming. Food is often used as a crutch to get through stressful times. But no matter how rushed or tired you feel, setting aside time for rest is essential to your goal of a healthy spirit, mind, and body.

God understood the importance of rest for Himself and His people, and He ordered weekly rest in one of the Ten Commandments: "For in six days the LORD made the heavens and the earth, the sea, and all

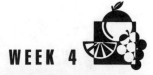

that is in them, and rested the seventh day. Therefore the LORD blessed the Sabbath day and hallowed it" (Ex. 20:11).

Perhaps you avoid rest because feelings of loneliness, anxiety, depression, or insecurity arise. Staying constantly busy is one way to avoid feeling. If you define your worth by your accomplishments, your sense of esteem and worth may fall when you stop performing and rest.

God created you in His image. You are a child of God, an heir of God, and when you experience the full meaning of that, you will understand you do not need to earn your worth by works. You can stop harming your health and relationships with God and others by overperforming. Jesus said, "Come to Me, all you who labor and are heavy laden, and I will give you rest" (Matt. 11:28).

When uncomfortable feelings arise, identify and try to resolve them rather than working nonstop or turning to food. Search your mind to determine their source. Are you trying to accomplish something or avoid something? Pinpointing a problem will allow you to develop a plan to solve it and not resort to self-destructive behavior.

Resisting change is natural, and rearranging your schedules and habits will require effort on your part. However, rest is such an important part of life, God mandated it. And it is an integral part of the Gentle Eating formula. The psalmist declared,

> I will both lie down in peace, and sleep;
> For You alone, O LORD, make me dwell in safety (Ps. 4:8).

You need sufficient rest to stay in balance, and as the Lord set the day aside for rest, you must plan for quiet time. Periods of relaxation will also help protect your immune system and increase mental functioning. Staying rested will reduce your desire to grab high-calorie snacks for a quick charge.

Daily rest allows for fellowship with the Lord and provides a break from the day's activities. And He said, "My presence will go with you, and I will give you rest" (Ex. 33:14).

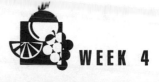

WEEK 4

Receiving God's Love and Comfort

You never have reason to doubt God's love for you. God gave a precious gift beyond price to you: He gave His only Son for your salvation. God's tremendous love for you is evident: "For God so loved the world that He gave His only begotten Son, that whoever believes in Him should not perish but have everlasting life" (John 3:16).

EXERCISE

1. What feelings arise when you ponder God's supreme act of love: giving His only Son for your salvation?

_____

_____

2. Do you acknowledge God's great love for you? In what ways?

_____

_____

3. Do you have beliefs and feelings that prevent you from accepting and basking in God's love?

_____

_____

Seeing God, Your Father, Through New Eyes

Paul wrote, "Long ago, even before he made the world, God chose us to be his very own, through what Christ would do for us; he decided then to make us holy in his eyes, without a single fault" (Eph. 1:4 TLB). God sees you through eyes of love, and there could be no greater show of His love than the giving of His Son so you might have eternal life. Learn to see God, your Father, through new eyes. Draw comfort and strength from His love and power when you feel hopeless and alone: "I can do all things through Christ who strengthens me" (Phil. 4:13).

What a wonderful God you have! He is the source of every mercy and the One who strengthens you in hardships and trials. And why does He do this? So that when others are troubled, needing your sympathy and encouragement, you can pass on to them the same help and comfort God has given you:

> Blessed be the God and Father of our Lord Jesus Christ, the Father of mercies and God of all comfort, who comforts us in all our tribulation, that we may be able to comfort those who are in any trouble, with the comfort with which we ourselves are comforted by God (2 Cor. 1:3–4).

EXERCISE

1. Do you sometimes feel God can't love you? Why?

_____

_____

_____

2. Scripture tells you, "Nor height nor depth, nor any other created thing, shall be able to separate us from the love of God which is in Christ Jesus our Lord" (Rom. 8:39). Study this passage and identify others you can seek out who reaffirm nothing has the power to stand between you and God.

_____

_____

_____

3. Your views of God might have been influenced by many sources. Can you name any of those sources?

_____

_____

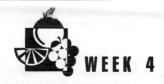

4. How do your views of God differ from the views of your family and friends?

_____

_____

_____

Do you close your heart and mind to avoid getting closer to God? God is patient, and He will wait for you to ask Him into your heart and life. Remember, you don't have to earn it. The price has been paid.

If you sometimes feel that your life is broken beyond repair, reflect on these passages:

> He heals the brokenhearted
> And binds up their wounds (Ps. 147:3).

> The LORD is near to those who have a broken heart,
> And saves such as have a contrite spirit (Ps. 34:18).

> Sing, O heavens!
> Be joyful, O earth!
> And break out in singing, O mountains!
> For the LORD has comforted His people,
> And will have mercy on His afflicted (Isa. 49:13).

Lord, I offer daily prayers of thanksgiving for Your love and encouragement as I seek to become a new person and leave old struggles and unhealthy choices behind. I acknowledge You as Lord of my life and feel secure in the knowledge that I am a child of God. I pray for Your aid as I make changes in my life that will bring me greater hope, peace, joy, and health. Thank You for showing me that all things are possible if only I put my trust and faith in You. As I face each new day, protect and shield me from all harm. Light my pathway today and every day. Amen.

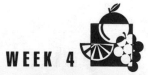

THINKING:
"Should" and "Shouldn't" Statements

Using "shoulds" and "shouldn'ts" to motivate yourself to lose weight often results in rebellious feelings and bingeing; overeating and guilt can quickly follow. When you fall short of your expectations (e.g., "I should have lost more weight by now"), you may experience disappointment, shame, and guilt. If you have been stung by past experiences with rejection and humiliation because you were overweight, you may have developed patterns of rebelliousness, anger, hypersensitivity, and difficulty with authority figures. Telling yourself no or you should or shouldn't eat something may trigger these negative feelings.

Learn to tell yourself, I can have anything I want to eat. Then take responsibility for your decision and go on from there.

EXERCISE

1. Record any occurrences of shoulds and shouldn'ts in your Thought Record.

2. How have shoulds and shouldn'ts controlled your life?

_____

_____

_____

3. What impact do "should" and "shouldn't" statements have on your eating behavior?

_____

_____

 **WEEK 4**

Labeling

Instead of saying, "I made a mistake and ate the wrong things," you label yourself: "I'm a pig, a loser." Labeling is an extreme form of overgeneralization. Rather than describing your behavior, "I don't want to exercise," you attach an emotionally loaded negative label to yourself: "I'm such a lazy slob!" You tell yourself, "I'm a failure," rather than, "I made a mistake." The fact is, your total self cannot equal any one thing.

Negative labels attack your self-worth and lead to feelings of depression, which could spark self-defeating behaviors. Learn to stay gentle with yourself, and you can and will develop positive behaviors that will enhance your life. Massage your feelings with kind thoughts.

EXERCISE

1. Record instances of negative labeling in your Thought Record.

2. What types of labels do you give yourself?

_____

_____

3. Where do you think these labels originated?

_____

_____

4. How does the way you label yourself make you feel?

_____

_____

5. What more gentle words can you say to yourself?

_____

_____

_____

EMOTIONAL:
The Road to Healing

You have been learning to identify the origin of pain, which can be embedded in your past, and how it may relate to your eating behavior. In this section you will learn to identify when and how your past experiences influence your present life. If you have food-related problems, you will discover there is a road to healing, and to travel it, you must resolve your past, get beyond your pain and hurts, and move forward.

Debbie was a thirty-five-year-old sales manager who had been in the Gentle Eating group for about a month. Debbie grew up in a family where sarcasm and put-downs were common. As an adult, she realized when she spent time around her family of origin, she was depressed for days afterward. Within minutes of her arrival at a family event, someone would say something negative to her. She would first experience a jab of hurt and then respond reflexively with a sarcastic comeback. The exchanges always ended in heated verbal arguments. During the interactions, Debbie said she felt fearful, helpless, and flustered— just as she had felt so many times before when she was growing up.

This reaction is termed *age regression*. It occurs when you feel like you did at an earlier age. You react emotionally, mentally, and defensively as you did then. On other occasions, with similar types of people and in similar circumstances, you might notice similar feelings. Perhaps you feel a sense of panic or shame after you become angry. As a child, you might never have learned how or been permitted to express your anger in a direct, assertive manner. The panic or shame might relate to a similar feeling you experienced at a younger age when you were angry. For example, as an adult, do you feel and react like you did as a child when an authority figure (perhaps, your boss) yells at you in anger?

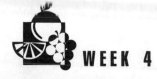

WEEK 4

Recognizing and Experiencing Your Feelings

You are no longer a child, so how do you stop age regression responses? How can you break free of the negative influences of your past? The first step is to become aware of the emotions. Next, notice the pattern of ongoing interaction. Who is usually involved? What do they say and do to cause you to feel negative emotions? Then, learn how to set boundaries with those involved and how to prepare for a given situation.

For instance, imagine you enter a social situation and you experience fear, hurt, or anger. Notice the feeling, but do not act on it. Instead, use calm, coping statements, such as, "Okay, take a deep breath; I can handle this"; or "I feel threatened and defensive, but all I need to do is focus on what to say or do to get through this. Everything will turn out okay."

Kay, another Gentle Eating group member, often felt a sense of unease around her younger sister, Diane. Unexpectedly, Diane would fly into a rage. The attacks were painfully similar to the rages their alcoholic father displayed when Kay and Diane were growing up. When Diane's anger was directed at her, Kay's stomach tensed up and she felt short of breath. Kay tried to cope with the stressful encounters, but she often felt verbally flayed by Diane and felt hurt and depressed for days.

Noticing this pattern and its frequency, Kay decided to protect herself by setting clear boundaries with Diane. As difficult as it was for her, Kay decided not to spend long periods of time with Diane. When Diane's raging started, Kay calmed herself and immediately left the scene; she did not remain involved in the combative verbal exchanges.

At times, you may not be able to leave the situation, but you can rehearse a protective response. You do not have to react or behave like a child victim, and you no longer need to remain silent when you are being verbally and emotionally abused.

Andrea, age forty-one, had to call and cancel her daughter's horse riding lesson. Chris, the woman in charge, was usually cross and rude. Andrea got a sick feeling just thinking about having to talk to Chris. She noticed a panicky feeling as if she was about to be scolded or attacked. Pondering on it, Andrea realized that she experienced a sense of shame when Chris spoke to her. Andrea felt that she had done something wrong or was bad.

Andrea's protective response plan included imagining Chris's cross or rude response and the feelings that Andrea then experienced as a result of the exchange. She practiced coping with the feelings by trying to stay calm, physically and mentally. She used positive coping statements that kept her grounded. When the usual feelings of fear and anxiety came up, her self-statements included, "Just stay focused. You're okay. The request is reasonable. If she doesn't like it, it's her problem. Your panic and fear are unfounded. Watch how well you handle the situation. That's it. Just speak directly and don't overapologize. You haven't done anything wrong."

The next time Andrea called to cancel a lesson, Chris remarked sarcastically, "I thought your daughter was serious about riding." Andrea fought the urge to defend herself and simply said, "I would like to keep her appointment next week." You can't control people like Chris; all you can do is strive to keep a clear head and stay calm. Notice the feelings that come up, label them, and learn to protect your feelings.

When dealing with insulting relatives, let them know if they continue that type of behavior, you will not remain in their presence. It is a harsh remedy, but it is a measure that works. Do not hesitate to use it if you have tried more gentle methods that have been ignored. You will immediately notice a feeling of relief and inner peace.

EXERCISE

1. Think of a situation in which you react emotionally similar to the way you did when you were a child. What is the situation? What people are involved?

_____

_____

_____

WEEK 4

2. What feelings come up?

_____

_____

_____

3. What can you say or do to stay in the present and remain task oriented?

_____

_____

_____

4. What plan can you devise and start to practice today?

_____

_____

_____

5. Where will you get this training?

_____

_____

_____

6. When and with whom will you practice your plan?

_____

_____

_____

How Your Past Influences Your Eating Behavior

A permanent move from the past to the present requires that you learn new reactions to people and situations that trigger old feelings. For example, growing up with critical parents or caregivers might cause you as an adult to overreact to perceived criticism from others. A critical comment directed to you as an adult might trigger a similar feeling you experienced as a child of being put down and not respected. This is a form of age regression. If someone berates you, the incident might bring up similar feelings of fear you experienced as a child. Age regression causes problems because childlike reactions are not adaptive for adult life.

EXERCISE 1

Write down patterns of age regression you have experienced as an adult. To understand the patterns, you may need to observe and record your feelings for a few days as you interact with difficult people in your life. Notice, for instance, whether you feel guilty when you think about asking or ask someone for help. This might suggest that you experience a feeling of shame (e.g., "I'm not worth it, I'm bad, different . . .") similar to one you had while growing up. Can you determine the source of this feeling?

Age regressed feelings: _____
_____ .

Experienced with (who was present?): _____
_____ .

Possible childhood origin: _____
_____ .

EXERCISE 2

Reflect on and write about the following experiences and how they may relate to your adult life.

1. Did you receive positive attention, special recognition, or praise for the adult roles you took on as a child?

_____

WEEK 4

2. If you answered yes, in what ways?

_____

_____

3. Was that the main or only way you received positive attention in your family?

_____

4. If you answered yes, how do you feel as you reflect on that reality now?

_____

_____

Family Times

EXERCISE

What was it like living with your family? Reflect on memories revolving around family times and write down your recollections.

When I came home from school, I remember _____

_____

_____.

When I returned home, the person who was there to meet me was _____

_____.

Being at home felt like _____

_____

_____.

Sitting together with the family in the evenings was _____

_____.

I often felt (anger, alone, anxious, on guard) _____

_____ .

Sitting together at the dinner table was _____

_____

_____ .

Going to bed at night, I remember feeling _____

_____

_____

If it could be different, I wish bedtime had been like this: _____

_____

_____ .

When I woke up in the mornings, I remember _____

_____

_____

Review your answers and think about possible connections with your use of food when you experience certain emotions. For example, one group member felt most secure in bed. She had come to associate food with security and often felt most secure (i.e., sheltered from her fears) when eating in bed.

Guilt and Shame

Guilt is a feeling you have when you sense that you have done something wrong. If you have healthy social skills, you probably develop a feeling of guilt when you have behaved in a manner that conflicts with your moral or ethical codes. Feelings of guilt are often followed by a feeling of sadness, which causes you to change your behavior. Ideally, guilt feelings are resolved by making amends or remedying the offense. Unresolved guilt can lead to a chronic sense of being bad. Lowered

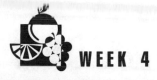

WEEK 4

self-esteem, depression, and even self-hatred can result. Unresolved guilt may be engendered by family members or brought on by a deep-seated sense of shame.

Whereas guilt is the feeling that "you did something wrong," shame is the feeling or belief that "you are something wrong," that you are defective or bad in some way. Since guilt is something you do, you can change it. Shame is not a behavior to be changed, but an enduring condition of badness or defectiveness, something you perceive you are. How do you develop a sense of shame? Parents or caregivers, teachers, and persons in authority collectively can contribute to your sense of shame with a barrage of negative messages and reprimands. Perhaps you grew up hearing messages like these: "You should be ashamed of yourself!" "How could you do such a thing?" "Is that the best you can do?" "What kind of boy or girl would do that?" Basically, the message is, "You're bad"; "You're not good enough"; or "No good person would do that."

Children are quick to believe the words of parents or caregivers, teachers, and persons in authority, especially when the words are delivered with intense emotion and perceived disgust. When children hear these hurtful words from people they idealize and depend upon, they internalize the words and believe them to be true. Shame can also result from erroneous conclusions children make (for example, they are "dummies" because they do not do well in reading or math, or their parents' divorce was their fault).

Young children are also shamed when they are scolded or put down for expressing how they feel. Parents or caregivers or others may deliver chastising statements:

- "Don't be such a baby!"
- "Dive in, it's not that cold!"
- "Oh, stop crying. She didn't hit you that hard!"
- "That's kindergarten stuff. I can't believe you can't do it!"

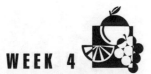

These statements can contribute to the erosion of the true self of children. To survive or gain approval, they cut themselves off from their feelings. They lose touch with the true self and how they really feel. They learn to suppress what they think and feel. They develop a false self.

Mapping the Path to Emotional Wholeness

If you have not done so, set aside some time to get to know the real you. One starting point is to note what feelings come up as you think about playing. Not just the word *playing*, but imagine yourself participating in acts of play. The concept of enjoying fun and games may seem remote. Perhaps when you were a child, playtime was a luxury you never knew. Maybe you had to use all of your energy just to survive in your family. In an extreme case, your family life might have been chaotic, or you never knew when a parent or caregiver would break into a rage or be drunk. Perhaps your perfectionist, high-achieving, workaholic tendencies do not permit play. Recapturing your desire and ability to play is part of developing into a whole person. Experiencing the exhilaration of carefree play requires that you reclaim a part of your child-self you may have disowned.

EXERCISE

If the idea of play seems too foreign to you, try doing some of the following activities. As you do these activities, notice what feelings come up and record them (e.g., guilt, fear, anxiety, embarrassment, joy, exhilaration).

1. Go to a park and start swinging.

_____

2. Buy a coloring book and crayons and spend an hour coloring.

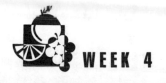

WEEK 4

3. Hold a doll and pretend to feed it.

4. Jump rope.

5. Roller-skate.

6. Sing a child's song.

7. Skip along.

8. Attend a children's movie.

Family Mealtimes

EXERCISE

Thinking back to your childhood, evaluate your family mealtime experiences.

1. Who was usually at the dining table?

2. What types of discussions were held?

3. How did you feel sitting at the table with each of those present?

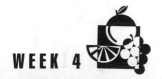

4. How did your early mealtime experiences influence your eating behavior?

_____

_____

Praise or Put-Downs?

A child hears positive affirming versus negative judgmental statements from parents or caregivers at a ratio of about one to four. Many parents or caregivers are unaware of put-down remarks they make. They often do not hear what children hear, and they do not understand the negativity ensconced in comments such as, "Now, why did you do that?" or in directive statements such as, "Stop doing that! Come and put your things away this minute!"

Negative overt or subtle messages become deeply ingrained in your subconscious and help lay the foundation for your self-image. Usually, you see yourself as your parents or caregivers see you. You learn who you are from their words and actions. You learn to think you are okay or not okay, or lovable or unlovable, from what they said or did not say, did or did not do.

EXERCISE 1

1. What positive messages did your parents or caregivers communicate to you? (Focus on those messages while you learn to deal with and cast aside the negative messages.)

_____

_____

2. What negative messages did your parents or caregivers communicate to you?

_____

_____

WEEK 4

3. What negative words were spoken or what negative actions were taken by your parents or caregivers in relation to food (e.g., when to eat, what to eat, how much to eat)?

_____

_____

4. What, if anything, did your parents or caregivers negatively communicate about your body's size or shape?

_____

_____

5. How did subtle or overt words or actions by your parents or caregivers influence the development of your body image?

_____

_____

_____

Sometimes parents or caregivers and other adults say the "right" words, but some hidden message or meaning is attached. For example, Sue's mother would seemingly defend Sue when her siblings teased about her weight. But her mother would say things like, "Sue is a big girl," or "Sue has a big appetite; we all have our battles to fight." Sue felt ambivalent about her mother's comments. Not until she became an adult did she realize why she felt anger toward her mother in relation to her weight.

EXERCISE 2

1. When you were growing up, what hidden messages did you hear about your weight or body size?

_____

_____

_____

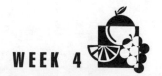

WEEK 4

2. Who said these things?

_____

3. What, if any, lasting impression did these words make?

_____

PHYSICAL:
Trimming the Fat

Here are the top ten sources of calories in the U.S. diet:

1. White bread, rolls
2. Doughnuts, cookies, cakes
3. Alcoholic beverages
4. Whole milk
5. Hamburgers, cheeseburgers, etc.
6. Beefsteaks, roasts
7. Soft drinks
8. Hot dogs, ham, lunch meat
9. Eggs
10. Fries, chips

Since 1985, when that survey was published in *The American Journal of Epidemiology,* hundreds of lower-calorie products have been introduced into the marketplace. You have many choices as you shop for fat busters.

We make no recommendation about whether or not you eat meat since that is a highly personal choice. Nor do we recommend particular products. The following excerpt from a major food chain publication dated March 1996 is included only to show comparative information on a relatively new product in the U.S.:

You'll find ostrich . . . in a variety of cuts including steaks, ground meat and Italian sausage.

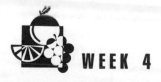

WEEK 4

Ostrich Vs. Beef and Chicken

Per 3 oz. portion	Fat	Calories	Cholesterol
Ostrich (Prime)	2 g.	97	58 mg.
Beef (Eye of Round)	6 g.	230	74 mg.
Chicken Breast (Skinless)	3 g.	140	73 mg.

Adopt a Slow, Get-Used-to-It Method

As you gradually trim fat from your diet, you will notice lower-fat foods can be satisfying, and you will have more energy. For instance, if you have been drinking whole milk and begin drinking 2 percent milk, it may taste like water, but you will become more satisfied with it in time. If you choose to switch to 1 percent or skim milk, your initial reaction will probably be the same as it was when you originally chose to try 2 percent milk.

Milk provides a wide range of essential nutrients, including vitamin B and calcium, and milk is also a complete protein with all essential amino acids. Low-fat and skim milk both have a cholesterol-reducing effect. Low-fat and skim yogurt work to lower cholesterol even more.

Nevertheless, reports continue to be published relating to whether or not milk is good for adults. It is true that some individuals are what has been termed *lactose intolerant;* however, some products on the market address that matter. There are also milk substitutes, so review your options on a personal level and make your decisions based on your needs and preferences and, if applicable, your doctor's advice.

Though you may be skeptical initially, your body will adjust and crave healthier foods as it craved unhealthy foods. In the meantime, remember that a moderate amount of fat and sugar is okay. Just do not overindulge.

Track Calorie Savings

You can lose a pound in a week by cutting 500 calories a day, and though your loss goal may be much lower, this modest cutback translates into a fifty-two-pound loss in a year! You do this by looking for and taking advantage of calorie savings.

For comparison purposes, be mindful of the following: 1 ounce of chocolate contains 145 calories and 9 grams of fat and derives 56 percent of calories from fat; 1 cup of ice cream contains 270 calories and 14 grams of fat and derives 47 percent of calories from fat; and 1 tablespoon of butter, lard, margarine, mayonnaise, or vegetable oil contains 100 calories and 11 grams of fat and derives 100 percent of calories from fat. Giving up one small chocolate bar, one cup of ice cream, and one tablespoon of butter (or the equivalent) daily would push you past the 500-calorie goal.

Following are additional tips for calorie savings:

- When you prepare an omelet, use two egg whites with only one egg yolk for a savings of 65 calories.
- An eight-ounce apple has about 127 calories; eat a four-ounce apple and cut that calorie count in half!
- You can save 100 calories by having frozen yogurt in a sugar (not waffle) cone. For an even bigger saving, ask that your treat be served in a paper cup.
- For a breakfast treat under 170 calories, mix one-fourth cup toasted wheat germ, one-half cup skim milk, and one-half cup fresh berries (or other fresh fruit).
- A chicken bouillon cube contains only 6 calories per cup of broth. The cubes are small and easy to carry with you and are great for curbing appetites. (Follow instructions on the package or container.)
- Multigrain or sprouted breads are high in fiber, with about 2 grams and 75 calories per slice. When making sandwiches, use only one slice of bread; the fiber is filling and you have saved 75 calories.
- Consider turkey ham a cold-cut choice; it's 95 percent fat-free.
- Three and one-half ounces of water-packed tuna contain 28 grams of protein and only 127 calories.

Remember, fat has twice as many calories per gram as protein and carbohydrates

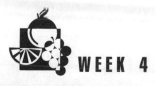

WEEK 4

When Shopping for Body Fuel, Be a Label Reader

It is almost a certainty you will choose to keep some higher-fat items in your food plan; after all, you do not want to be too stringent, or you risk going off your program in frustration. Try to serve these items less often, and allow yourself smaller portions. Learn to plan the majority of your menus concentrating on foods lower in fat.

Pay special attention to product labels showing low-fat and low-calorie to determine percentages and sources of fat. (A fat-finding formula is provided later on.) This may be confusing at first, but your efforts will be rewarded as you enjoy a healthier lifestyle. Stick with your plan—label reading will become less time consuming, and you will have the satisfaction of knowing what fuel you are giving your body.

These definitions may be helpful:

- Reduced fat: 25 percent less fat than the original product
- Lean: less than 10 grams of fat per 100 grams
- Extra lean: less than 5 grams of fat per 100 grams
- Low-calorie: 40 calories or less per serving
- Low-fat: 3 grams of fat or less per serving
- Fat-free: less than 0.5 gram of fat per serving
- Light or lite: one-third fewer calories, one-half the fat, or one-half the sodium of the original product

Good Fat Versus Bad Fat

Many nutritionists agree that fat from plants, rather than from animal sources, is healthier for your body. Saturated fat (lard and butter) comes from animal products and is generally in solid form at room temperature. Unsaturated fat (vegetable oil) is liquid at room temperature. Polyunsaturated fats are in oils such as sesame, corn, sunflower, safflower, and soybean. Olive and canola oils are monounsaturated fats and are healthier alternatives of fats.

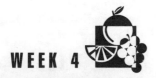

WEEK 4

Monounsaturated fats help lower health-threatening cholesterol levels derived from low-density lipoprotein, or LDL. High-density lipoprotein, or HDL, cholesterol is beneficial to your body and helps prevent and fight heart disease.

If you eat meat, slowly reduce your consumption of red meat, and eat turkey, chicken, and fish more often than beef. Always eat lean, thoroughly cooked cuts of meat.

The Fat-Finding Formula

To determine your daily fat intake, use the following formula. Each gram of fat has 9 calories. If you eat a 4-ounce portion of beef with 400 total calories and 20 grams of fat, multiply grams of fat times calories, which equals 180. The ratio of 180/400 yields percentage of fat calories: 45 percent. Almost half the calories in that small portion of meat are derived from fat. By contrast, a can of vegetable soup has 90 calories and 2 grams of fat, showing 20 percent of calories from fat.

EXERCISE

List several favorite foods and compute percentage of fat grams in each product. Below each food listed, name a lower-fat substitute you would consider eating. Compute the percentage of fat grams in each alternative. Contrast your findings.

Food: _____   % Fat Grams: _____
Substitute: _____   % Fat Grams: _____

Food: _____   % Fat Grams: _____
Substitute: _____   % Fat Grams: _____

Food: _____   % Fat Grams: _____
Substitute: _____   % Fat Grams: _____

Food: _____   % Fat Grams: _____
Substitute: _____   % Fat Grams: _____

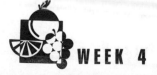

WEEK 4

Consuming excessive calories derived from fat compromises your health and puts you at risk for the following leading causes of disease and death:

- High LDL cholesterol
- Stroke
- Heart disease
- Cancer
- Gall bladder disease
- High blood pressure

A report in the *Archives of Ophthalmology* has highlighted another serious health concern. A five-year study of eighteen thousand healthy physicians yielded this disturbing conclusion: Scientists found that the heaviest among the subjects were more than twice as likely as doctors of normal weight to develop cataracts. Cataracts are the leading cause of blindness worldwide, but they are potentially preventable. The bottom line, then, is this: Being overweight appears to sharply raise your chances of developing cataracts and provides another important reason to take STEPs to manage your weight by making gradual and lasting changes in your dietary habits.

Carbohydrates give you energy, proteins build a strong, healthy body, and excess fat makes you gain weight! Your body stores fat more readily than proteins or carbohydrates, and in the U.S., much of the fat consumed comes from meat, dairy products, and oils. Learn to prepare favorite foods utilizing lower-fat methods, some of which are suggested in this workbook. You will be able to find many others in food sections of daily newspapers, magazines, cookbooks, and pamphlets at your local supermarkets. Also, try to eat protein alternatives to high-fat meat.

Were You Born with a Sweet Tooth?

Do you have a natural preference for sweet-tasting foods? Almost all of us do. But consuming large amounts of high-fat, high-sugar foods low in nutrition is the formula for poor health and high weight.

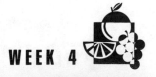

A moderate amount of sugar daily will not throw your systems off balance. However, high doses of sugar cause a rise in blood sugar levels, which then drop drastically. A sudden drop in blood sugar activates a plunge in mood and sharp increase in appetite. Try to keep your blood sugar levels constant by eating fruits and other carbohydrates that process sugar more slowly. Overeating in any food category will disrupt your body's systems.

Calories: To Count or Not to Count?

Many chronic dieters have practically memorized calorie books, and they can tell you how many calories are in each type of food. But relying solely on counting calories apparently has not helped the approximately 90 to 95 percent of dieters who regain weight. A basic knowledge of calories is important and useful in your weight management program; however, obsessive concern about how many calories each bit of food contains may contribute to the anxiety-deprivation-binge cycle described earlier. So, pay attention to all of the STEPs, and do not focus or rely on one method such as calorie counting.

Calories Do Not Come Out of Thin Air!

Calories are fuel: a measure of energy. There is nothing mysterious about them. Some nutritionists claim that calories are calories, dismissing the fact that your body burns low-fat, high-bulk carbohydrates more efficiently. Therefore, knowing the *source* of your calories can be a valuable weight management tool.

EXERCISE

List some of the types of food you now eat and whether they are a carbohydrate, protein, or fat source. Compute the percentage of calories derived from fat grams.

WEEK 4

Food	Food Source	Percentage of Calories from Fat*
1.		
2.		
3.		
4.		
5.		

*Use the fat-finding formula.

Proteins: Only a Small Part of the Picture

If you have followed low-fat, high-protein diets and are still seeking to solve your weight management problem, you have probably realized that such a lopsided approach will not succeed in the long term.

Protein is an essential body builder; new muscle, bones, skin, and hair cells depend on protein. Protein also regulates metabolism, body fluids, and other critical body functions. But protein is only part of the picture. Without sufficient carbohydrates, protein and fat are used for fuel, and when protein is depleted, it is not readily available for other vital body needs.

When you adhere to a high-protein, low-carbohydrate, and low-fat diet, ketosis (a waste product) becomes unbalanced and causes your body to eliminate excessive amounts of water, resulting in quick weight loss. But ketosis will soon return, and you will register a weight gain.

Protein is either used by your body or eliminated; it is not stored. It must be replaced daily. For that reason, you should eat small amounts of protein at each meal.

How much protein do you really need daily? Very little! Nutritionists and health experts generally recommend that only 20 percent of your daily calories come from protein. Surveys reveal Americans generally consume more than three times that amount. (For comparison: a six-ounce can of tuna provides more than the suggested daily portion

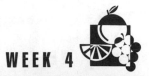

of protein.) Ideally, small amounts of protein should be consumed throughout the day rather than a large amount at one sitting. Protein is much easier to digest in small quantities. Inundating your body with a six- or eight-ounce steak, together with a potato, sour cream, and/or butter, taxes your digestive system. Research has shown excess meat may take up to thirty hours to digest in your intestines.

Sources of Protein

Protein that has been described as complete comes from animal sources. However, legumes and beans, combined with grains or seeds, are also good sources of protein. If weight management is a concern, you should be aware of fat content in various proteins. Fat in beef consumed in excessive amounts may be partly responsible for heart disease and several types of cancer. Practicing moderation in all food categories will lead to overall better health.

EXERCISE

Review the following list of foods rich in protein. To learn the amount of fat each contains, read packaging labels or grocery store flyers, books, newspaper articles, or magazine articles. This information will aid you in meal planning for a balanced menu. (Research as many as you choose; it is not necessary to spend a lot of time if you cannot readily find the information.)

Protein Source	Amount of Fat	Eaten at Which Meal
Egg (especially egg whites)		
Milk (low-fat/ nonfat)		
Yogurt (low in sugar)		

WEEK 4

Protein Source	Amount of Fat	Eaten at Which Meal
Low-fat/nonfat cream cheese		
Low-fat/nonfat cottage cheese		
Mozzarella cheese (or other skim milk cheese or cheese product)		
Seafood (especially tuna in water)		
Poultry, chicken, turkey (especially white meat)		
Cornish game hens		
Lean, trimmed pork, lamb, and beef		
Veal		
Legumes (to be eaten with grains/seeds):		
Beans		
Lentils		
Red beans		
Split peas		
Soybeans		
Kidney beans		
Black-eyed peas		
Northern beans		
Lima beans		
Navy beans		
Garbanzo (low-salt) beans		

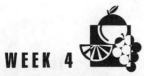

WEEK 4

Protein Source	Amount of Fat	Eaten at Which Meal
Legumes:		
Black beans		
Peanuts and pea-nut butter (low salt)		
Combine legumes with:		
Sunflower seeds		
Sesame seeds		
Pumpkin seeds		
Rice (preferably brown)		
Wheat (bread)		
Oats (breads, muffins)		
Corn (tortillas, muffins)		

Carbohydrates

Fad diets, myths, and misinformation have given carbohydrates an undeserved bad reputation nutritionally. Carbohydrates are another part of the picture, and you need to include simple and complex carbohydrates in your daily meal plans. You do not need to consume large amounts of carbohydrates. Unlike proteins, unused carbohydrates are stored as fat and remain in that form unless burned as fuel.

Compared to protein, carbohydrates are a more efficient source of energy. Your body is forced to work harder when it has to use protein for fuel.

Vegetables are excellent sources of carbohydrates, have relatively few calories, and contain fiber that curbs appetite for long periods of time. (Vegetables also contain an abundance of phytochemicals, which are potent compounds giving color, flavor, and aroma. For example, the orange pigment in sweet potatoes and carrots in beta-carotene,

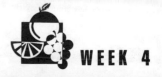

WEEK 4

which the body converts to vitamin A. These compounds help protect us from cancer, heart disease, and diabetes.)

Carbohydrates are categorized either as simple or as complex. Simple carbohydrates include the following:

- Fruits (all kinds)
- Vegetables ("nonstarchy"):

Zucchini	Red beets
Celery	Broccoli
Greens	Cauliflower
Mushrooms	Asparagus

Complex carbohydrates include the following:

- Grains:

Cereals	Pasta
Bread	Rice
Oats	Crackers
Barley	

- Vegetables ("starchy"):

Lima beans	Corn
Black-eyed peas	Winter squash
Turnips	Sweet and white potatoes

An average potato has only one hundred calories and so many essential nutrients that potatoes are the primary food staple in many countries. They are a rich source of carbohydrates and should not be viewed as forbidden. (High-calorie toppings, however, should be used sparingly if at all!)

Homeostasis: A Different Balancing Act

According to *Webster's II New Riverside University Dictionary*, equilibrium is "A condition in which all acting influences are canceled by others, resulting in a stable, balanced, or unchanging system." *Homeostasis* is

"A state of physiological equilibrium produced by a balance of functions and chemical composition within an organism."

Your body is designed to maintain homeostasis between different but related functions, and it has regulators or messengers to tell you when something is out of balance. When you repeatedly ignore your body's signals, your physiology becomes out of kilter, and organs and bodily functions deteriorate and break down.

This happens during chronic stress; your heart is taxed because it is overworked. Gastritis often develops, the intestines become inflamed and irritated, and you experience chronic diarrhea. Similarly, when you rob your body of important carbohydrates, proteins, vitamins, minerals, electrolytes, and so on, your body's ability to maintain internal balance is at risk. Additionally, signals for hunger or fullness are compromised or lost.

Your body was designed and created by God according to a system of balance. Daily consuming adequate amounts of food at proper intervals allows your body to function normally—to remain in balance. When nutritional elements are excluded, your body's attempts to regulate itself fail. Your vital organs become stressed; ultimately, they are damaged.

Bulk Foods

Foods high in fiber are important to weight management. Aside from other health benefits, high-fiber foods tend to push food through your intestines, eliminating more calories and allowing less fat to be absorbed into the digestive system. Approximately thirty grams of fiber are recommended in your daily food intake.

When you think of fiber, do you immediately think of bran? Bran is an excellent source of fiber, but in natural form its taste has not generated favorable comments. (That is, the taste leaves a lot to be desired!) Variety is the key to avoiding fiber burnout, and other very good sources of fiber include uncooked fruits, raw vegetables, whole grain cereals and breads. One-half cup of cooked spinach has more fiber than an equivalent amount of cooked cauliflower or beans, or an apple.

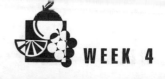

WEEK 4

How much fiber does a child need? "The right amount—in grams—is the child's age plus five. For example, a 10-year-old would need 15 grams per day. There are three or four grams of fiber in a serving of fruit, two or three grams in a ½ cup of veggies and one to five grams in a bowl of fiber-rich cereal. Adults 20 and older need 25 to 35 grams per day" *(Bottom Line Personal).*

As you accumulate more low-fat, high-fiber recipes, make it a habit to list necessary ingredients on the recipe card. This is a convenient method of having much of your shopping list prepared in advance. (Remember to take along the list when you shop!)

EXERCISE

1. List high-fiber foods you now use.

_____

_____

_____

2. List several additional fiber sources you will try.

_____

_____

_____

Whole—A Lot Better:

Vitamins Lost When Whole Wheat Is Refined*

Percent	Vitamin	Percent	Vitamin
86%	Vitamin E	70%	Vitamin B-6
81%	Niacin	67%	Folic Acid
80%	Riboflavin	50%	Pantothenic Acid
77%	Thiamin		

*H. A. Shroeder, *The Trace Elements and Man* (Old Greenwich, Conn.: Devin-Adair, 1973) 57.

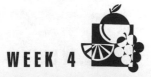

PROGRESS CHART

Check all that apply.

Spiritual Changes

___ Had at least a fifteen-minute daily quiet time.

___ Memorized a Bible verse.

___ Met with midweek church group.

___ Went to church services.

___ Prayed.

___ Felt a little closer to the Lord.

___ Expressed true feelings to God.

___ Honestly evaluated my relationship with God.

Thinking Changes

___ Recognized and recorded a distorted thought.

___ Experienced change in how I view myself.

___ Experienced change in how I thought about a situation.

___ Was able to develop more accurate/balanced view of person, event, etc.

Emotional Changes

___ Recorded my feelings.

___ Evaluated feelings before eating.

___ Expressed feelings in appropriate manner.

___ Noticed impact a person, place, or event had on my urge to eat.

___ Identified a past trauma or hurt.

___ Sought support from a trusted person.

___ Expressed hurt or pain in appropriate way.

___ Noticed how past hurt was related to urge to eat.

___ Worked on a stage of grief.

___ Noticed a change in level of a negative emotion.

___ Noticed a different reaction to person, place, or event that used to evoke emotional upset.

___ Implemented clear, personal emotional boundaries.

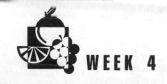

WEEK 4

PROGRESS CHART

Check all that apply.

Physical/Behavioral Changes

___ Charted my eating patterns.

___ Did workbook exercises.

___ Tried a new low-fat recipe.

___ Performed at least ten minutes of physical activity.

___ Listened to or watched ten to twenty minutes of a relaxation tape (audio or video).

___ Took at least fifteen minutes for myself.

___ Left some food on my plate.

___ Set a nice table with special touches: flowers, tablecloth, candles; listened to soothing music during mealtime; used special dishes.

___ Went shopping when not hungry.

___ Ate intended portions and stopped.

___ Rated hunger level before and after meals.

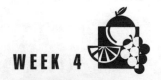

WEEK 4

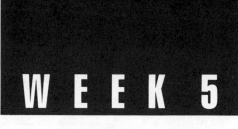

WEEK 5

SPIRITUAL:
Cast Off the Burden
of Old Grief, Gripes,
and Grudges

■ If you are carrying around old grief, gripes, and grudges, you are probably so burdened that healthy changes in your life may take longer. Ask God's help in setting aside this baggage and moving your life forward. It is never too late or too early to take a path that will lead to better health.

Begin each day by reminding yourself: "This is a new day, and I am a new person." You may want to memorize this: "Be renewed in the spirit of your mind" (Eph. 4:23).

Depend on a close relationship with God in all matters so that peace and comfort will be with you daily. Make sure there is no place for past hurts, disappointments, or failures in your renewed life. Ask God's help in casting off these burdens. The load is too heavy for you to bear and acts as a stumbling block to your spiritual growth and happiness. Think of things for which you should be grateful. Count your blessings.

EXERCISE

1. Do you expect unconditional love and regard from others because God gives both to you? Are these expectations realistic?

WEEK 5

_____
_____
_____

2. Do you often feel hurt or disappointed? Can you determine who or what caused such feelings?

_____
_____
_____

3. Do you need to make changes in your expectations? How will this help you cope?

_____
_____
_____

4. God is the most powerful source of strength you can call upon. Through prayer, tap into that source and make it a daily part of your life. Record what happens.

_____
_____
_____

5. Is there a stumbling block in your path keeping you from putting your absolute trust in God? (Make it a stepping-stone; go to Him in prayer, and nothing can keep you from experiencing God's deep and abiding love for you, His child.)

_____

Does Your Caring Nature Mask Codependency?

Are Christians more vulnerable than non-Christians to developing codependent behaviors? Codependency occurs when people put the

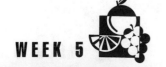

needs of others above their own. Codependents often attempt to gain self-esteem from being a helper or enabler of others. They may feel unduly responsible for the suffering of others and feel they have to fix it.

Codependents are overly concerned with pleasing others, often to the detriment of all concerned. This is especially true if codependent behavior enables someone to continue destructive behavior.

Be gentle with people who suffer and are in pain, offer prayers for God's intervention and help, but realize that you are not the ultimate answer to their problems; God is the answer. Direct people in need to God.

EXERCISE

1. In what way(s) do you relate to the discussion of codependency?

_____

_____

_____

2. Do you sometimes feel responsible when others are suffering or have problems? Do you feel compelled to fix it? (Understand that you do not have to ignore the plight of others. Offer to help in ways that will not tie you to each other in a codependent manner. Beyond that, pray with and for them; direct them to God, a source of power that surpasses all others.)

_____

_____

3. Can you think of ways in which you exhibit codependent behaviors?

_____

_____

_____

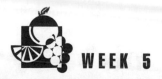

WEEK 5

4. Do you try to take on the problems of others as a way to gain acceptance? Give examples.

_____

_____

_____

5. Do you think that Christians may be more vulnerable than non-Christians to behaving codependently by rushing to help? Reflect on this, and try to determine when it is good to offer help (and what kind of help) and when it might not be beneficial.

_____

_____

_____

6. If your reflection shows that your codependency fosters irresponsibility, dysfunctionality, and lack of accountability on the part of another, think what God would have you do. Are you unknowingly keeping someone from turning to Him? (No matter how difficult it might seem, people must face their problems, take responsibility for their behavior, and make appropriate changes.)

_____

_____

_____

7. Read 1 Corinthians 10:23–33; 14:26–29. Do these passages help you understand the difference between pleasing others and helping others for unhealthy versus healthy reasons?

_____

Lord, Give Me Patience—Right Now Please!

Though in today's fast-paced world we would like to make that request, we understand the life of a Christian is not about quick fixes and instant gratification. It is a process, a way of life, a defined path

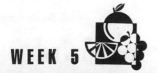

to follow, and it requires patience, understanding, and nurturing. Do not look for shortcuts; there are none.

This is also true for managing weight and maintaining emotional well-being. Both are processes that take time and effort. Be gentle with yourself and others, and rely on the Lord. It sounds like a contradiction in terms, but to achieve your goals, "slow and easy does it" is the fastest way and the lasting way.

Learning to think long term is part of your weight control process as well. Gently and gradually without undue stress, pursue your goals. If your goals are realistic, you will reach them. With God's help and your effort they are attainable.

EXERCISE

1. Do not become discouraged. List some of your achievements and focus on them.

_____

_____

_____

2. Be patient. Pray for guidance. Follow God's instructions. Search out Scriptures relating to your experiences and study them for guidance. Note which passages seem most helpful at present.

_____

_____

_____

With men it is impossible, but not with God (Mark 10:27).

Self-Control Versus Willpower

Ask yourself, Who's in charge of my life anyway? If you respond, I am, you need to examine your answer. Have faith that you must

WEEK 5

place God in charge of your life if you are to succeed. First, you must make an important distinction: Self-control is not willpower. Read Galatians 5:16–26 to understand the difference between willpower—something you try to do/not do on your own—and self-control—fruit you receive when you allow the Holy Spirit to work in your life.

You have probably heard it from many sources: "Attaining and maintaining an ideal weight require enormous willpower." That is not a true statement as you will learn by studying the distinction between willpower and self-control. Permanent weight management requires that you have realistic goals and become emotionally and spiritually healthy. And when you return food to its proper role of nourishing your body, you will eat normally.

In Galatians, Paul tells us to obey the Holy Spirit's instructions to do what we should do. As you stay connected to God, in prayer and communion with Him, you are more likely to hear the Holy Spirit. God will produce the fruits of love, joy, peace, patience, kindness, goodness, faithfulness, gentleness, and self-control in your life if you invite Him to work His will.

EXERCISE

1. Do you realize the difference between willpower and self-control? How can that distinction aid you in your weight management goals?

_____

_____

2. Pray to the Lord, "Thy will be done," and understand that through the power of the Holy Spirit you can gain self-control. List an instance where self-control would have made the difference in a good and bad ending.

_____

_____

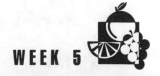

Lord, what a difference You have made in my life's journey! Patience and gentle changes in my lifestyle have made me realize that daily decisions, prayerfully made, are easier and I do not feel helpless or alone. I know You are with me always. Anxiety, which had often ruled my thoughts, has been banished and replaced by calm reason as I make healthier choices in my food selections and exercise habits. I place my faith and trust in You as I cast aside old ways of coping, which kept me from successfully managing my problems. I pray for You to strengthen me, for when I rely on my strength alone, I find it lacking, and I sometimes grow weak and weary before my tasks are completed. Amen.

THINKING:
Personalizing Blame

Personalizing blame occurs when you blame yourself for something, though you are not entirely responsible. Or you might blame others and overlook ways in which your attitudes and behaviors contribute to the problem. This error corresponds to a tendency of some dieters to attribute slips in their weight control programs to personal internal failings, such as a lack of willpower or a weak character.

Like other distortions, personalizing blame can leave you feeling guilty and bad about yourself. Instead, focus on behaviors and situations that make it difficult to stay with your program and think what you can do differently to ensure a positive outcome. Then do it!

EXERCISE

1. How do you personalize blame?

_____

_____

WEEK 5

2. How does this distorted thinking influence your eating behavior?

_____

_____

3. How can you view the situation less personally?

_____

_____

4. How can you get beyond assigning blame and learn to accept responsibility?

_____

_____

Catastrophizing

Catastrophizing refers to exaggerating the importance of things or making mountains out of molehills. Instead of thinking how to cope successfully after a mistake, you search your mind for the worst outcome imaginable and assume it lurks around every corner. For example, you look in a mirror, see you have gained weight, panic, and determine you are going to get fatter and fatter. Then you figuratively give the negativity wings, and it flies through your mind to conclude that you will be rejected, abandoned, and alone; no one will want you as a mate or companion. Feeling depressed and hopeless, you overeat to soothe the pain.

EXERCISE

1. In what general ways do you catastrophize?

_____

_____

2. How do you catastrophize regarding food and your eating habits?

_____

_____

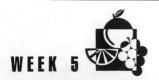

3. How does this thinking distortion lead to out-of-control eating behaviors?

_____

_____

_____

4. Record instances of catastrophizing when you think about losing weight and keeping it off.

_____

_____

_____

EMOTIONAL:
Moving Beyond Past
Loss and Pain

A loss is an event that can cause deep sadness or mental distress, and it occurs when you no longer have something you once had. A loss can also be something you felt you should have had but never did.

Losing a parent or caregiver through divorce or death, or never having had a father's or mother's love and companionship, can deeply affect your emotional development. In each instance, there is a loss, and the absence of a father or mother is a loss that many never stop grieving. When the loss is not grieved, loss is repressed and pushes for expression. The result is usually an unhealthy outlet, and a major unhealthy outlet is indulging in food binges as you seek comfort.

Playing Hide-and-Seek with Feelings

If you have repressed or hidden your feelings in the past, you need to learn to track, find, and release such feelings as you seek emotional wholeness. A first step to identifying the emotions you have kept inside.

153

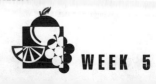 **WEEK 5**

EXERCISE

Check the feelings you seldom experience or you feel uncomfortable experiencing:

___ Joy	___ Spontaneity	___ Rage
___ Enthusiasm	___ Happiness	___ Relaxation
___ Compassion	___ Contentment	___ Peace
___ Empathy	___ Anger	___ Hurt
___ Sadness	___ Guilt	___ Fear
___ Security	___ Trust	___ Pride
___ Innocence	___ Tranquillity	

When Just a Band-Aid Won't Do

As you were growing up, perhaps you were unable to grieve your losses. Or maybe you did not consider your experiences as losses. If you determine you are experiencing unresolved grief, rather than medicate or attempt to avoid pain through food abuse or other self-destructive behavior, face and grieve the pain. If applicable, acknowledge the loss or absence of significant relationships during your life and the impact of the loss or absence on you. And let go of your unsuccessful ways of coping.

Though you may realize your familiar ways of coping are not working, you may be reluctant to change. But you need to examine your old behaviors, cast aside unworkable, self-defeating ones, and make beneficial changes. The changes might include these:

- Letting go of using food to contend with difficulties
- Learning to communicate instead of argue
- Learning to stop blaming others for your perceived lack of success

Grieving a loss is an essential emotional experience, and when there is unresolved grief, physical and psychological problems can develop.

Like other repressed emotions, unresolved grief is unexpressed energy, which can lead to chronic anxiety, anger, apprehension, depression, excessive guilt, or shame.

EXERCISE 1

For a moment, imagine your life as a train on a track pulling a line of boxcars. One of the boxcars is labeled "Repressed Feelings/Unresolved Grief," and it is partially filled. Wedged among the cargo are chronic anxiety, apprehension, and depression, and you can visualize other unwanted passengers waiting to hop aboard. Mentally unhook the boxcar. Leave it behind. Lighten the load. Continue your journey as you watch the boxcar fade from view.

EXERCISE 2

1. What losses do you need to grieve (e.g., loss of parent or caregiver because of divorce or death; never experiencing a close, loving relationship with your mother and/or your father)?

_____

_____

2. To what extent were you able to grieve your losses when they occurred? (For instance, "I wasn't able to talk to Mom about how I missed Dad, because she hated him. I just learned not to say anything.")

_____

_____

3. Healthy grieving requires that you talk about the experience and share it with a safe person. Identify person(s) you feel you can

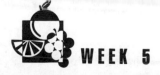

share your losses with (e.g., family member, friend, spouse, counselor, doctor, teacher).

_____

_____

4. Why are you not willing to go into individual therapy to work on losses?

_____

_____

5. Why are you considering going into individual therapy to work on losses?

_____

_____

EXERCISE 3

Check which, if any, of the following you consider personal losses:

___ Not having a happy, close family.

___ Not having healthy parents or caregivers.

___ Parents' or caregivers' separation or divorce.

___ Not having parents or caregivers who liked each other.

___ Not having parents or caregivers who loved each other.

___ Having to move and leave close friends and familiar surroundings.

___ Separation from siblings and stepsiblings.

___ Not having enough time with Mom or Dad because of too many siblings or a sibling with a disability.

___ Not being allowed to be afraid because of codependent role.

___ Not experiencing a significant part of my teen or young adult years because of involvement with an addiction.

___ Losing a favorite toy or special item.

___ Death of a relative or friend.

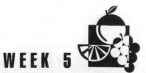

— Loss of true self (i.e., being forced into a role, unrealistic expectations, lack of encouragement).

— Aborted babies.

— Relationships that ended when I did not want them to end.

— Lack of good self-concept.

— Lack of healthy self-esteem.

Time Heals

As you try to come to terms with your loss, try to recognize where you are in the grieving process to determine what has been left undone. You may then be able to take positive steps toward a resolution and not remain stuck. For example, young children who have been abused often deny the pain of their abuse or blame themselves for what happened. Feeling they are protecting their parents or caregivers or others, they may stay in denial or stuck in depression, never reaching resolution or acceptance of what happened to them. Food and other addictions often serve as cover-ups for unresolved grief, and until the cover-ups are removed and the pain resolved, unhealthy behavior continues. Time heals, but first the wound must be cleansed.

The following is a brief narration you can transfer to a cassette tape if you choose. Get comfortable, close your eyes, and listen to your tape. Allow yourself to experience whatever comes up. If your mind wanders, gently bring yourself back to focus. After you finish listening, write down your thoughts and feelings.

Take a few comfortable breaths. Begin to feel your body relaxing—even just a little bit. From the top of your head all the way to the tips of your toes. See yourself with a backpack. Open it. Put into the backpack all of your losses and hurts. Put all other past issues that are blocking your emotional growth into the backpack. Add to the backpack all current matters that are troubling you, one by one: all the pain you have suffered, all the hurts that keep you from experiencing all that God has for you. When you feel you have put everything you wanted to into the backpack, close it. Put it on your

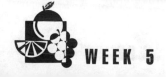

WEEK 5

back and see yourself walking down a lovely path in the woods. The temperature is exactly how you like it. Notice the beautiful surroundings: the gentle swaying of the green trees, the sunlight sparkling through the leaves. Hear the birds chirping. Feel the warm breeze on your face. Just ahead is an incline up a steep hill.

Going up the incline, you begin to feel the weight of the pack on your back. It's getting heavier and heavier against your shoulders and spine. With each step it feels like the backpack is a ton of bricks. Up ahead is a lovely meadow. You see a large red helium balloon with broad yellow stripes. There is a rope anchoring the balloon. Go over to the balloon and put your backpack next to the basket.

Open your backpack and pull out all of your hurts, losses, and disappointments, one by one. Put them into the basket of the balloon. There may be some losses or hurts that you aren't ready or able to give up. Leave them for now. When you are finished, untie the rope anchoring the balloon. Lie back on the grass and watch the balloon float up, up, and away. Notice how much better you feel. There is a sense of relief. Where in your body do you feel lighter and more peaceful? Continue watching the balloon drift away.

EXERCISE

1. What past hurts did you put in the backpack?

_____

_____

2. Which ones did you choose to keep for now?

_____

_____

3. What feelings came up for you during the narration?

_____

_____

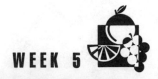

WEEK 5

An Unsent Letter—No Postage Required

Imagine back to when you were a young child. Write a letter to the parents or caregivers who hurt you as a child. In your letter, tell them how they hurt you and what effect it had on your life. You can also tell them what you needed from them but never got. Finally, tell them what you wished was different about your childhood and your relationship with them. Don't hold back. Write out all your feelings; this is a way to let negative feelings go.

It may serve your purpose to only imagine writing a letter. Find a quiet place, close your eyes, and vent your feelings through an imaginary letter first and reflect later to see how you feel about this method. For instance, do you feel you have made progress in getting it out of your system? You may want to repeat the exercise at another time to add a "P.S." But do not become obsessive; the goal is to leave negative thoughts and feelings behind.

In any event, *do not actually send a letter.* The objective is to release negative feelings you may harbor; it is not to hurt or punish others.

EXERCISE

1. What emotions came up for you as you wrote or imagined the letter (e.g., relief, disloyalty, anger, satisfaction)?

_____

_____

2. What positive actions can you take to enable you to release lingering negative feelings?

_____

_____

Should You Sever the Ties That Bind?

Inadequate or unfulfilled relationships with one or both parents, or your caregivers, might have left you feeling cheated and needy. Do you

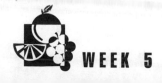

feel you keep running into a wall of rejection as you keep trying to gain acceptance, understanding, and love? Perhaps your parents or caregivers do not have the ability to change and give you what you need. Or though it may be an unhappy realization, they may not be able to comprehend those needs.

One step in accepting the loss of good relationships with your parents or caregivers is letting go of the emotional hold they have on you, literally severing the ties that bind. If you feel you have exhausted ways to reconcile your situation, stop setting yourself up for repeated hurt, and be willing to acknowledge the loss and start the healing process. Accept that the love, approval, acceptance, and understanding you seek are probably not going to come from that source. Search for healthy substitutes to counter the loss. Certainly, continue to pray for change, but turn the matter over to God. The ultimate plan is His.

You might want to write out a script and tape-record this. Sit across from someone you trust and feel safe with. Have the person hold one end of a rope and you hold the other, with the rope representing the ties you have to your parents or caregivers. The person holding the other end of the rope plays the role of the parents or caregivers, and you are yourself. Tell the parents or caregivers you are going to stop trying to get their approval, acceptance, love, and understanding. Let them know your feelings about your unmet needs. Tell them that you are going to stop trying, that you are now going to accept the reality of their limitations as parents or caregivers. Freely express your hurt, anger, sadness, and disappointment. When you have finished, let go of your end of the rope. You have taken the first step in letting go, surrendering to God what you have tried to, but cannot, change.

EXERCISE 1

1. My feelings that came up during this exercise were

_____

_____.

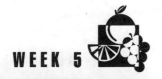

2. I was able to let go of

_____

_____.

3. I was not able to let go of

_____

_____.

4. I feel I am being blocked from letting go and moving on by

_____

_____.

5. I feel that taking the following steps will enable me to let go:

_____

_____.

6. I will do this (soon, this month, or when?)

_____

_____.

EXERCISE 2

List possible surrogate parents you can interact with to get your needs for approval, love, acceptance, and understanding met. Consider an older couple, other relatives, or close friends.

_____

_____

_____

Support Groups: To Join or Not to Join?

Letting go of the past and living in the present are often facilitated by interaction with people you consider safe. Creating or joining a support system is often a pivotal part of weight management programs. Gentle Eating group members report that going through this workbook in a group gave them added motivation, focus, and resolve to make small, gentle changes toward a healthier lifestyle. You may want to join a Gentle Eating group in your area, or you may want to start one. Visit a session and gauge your reaction. Or you may choose not to share your journey at this time. Do not place yourself in a situation in which you feel uncomfortable.

(Guides for setting up and conducting a Gentle Eating group are provided in Appendices A and B.)

Becoming an Overcomer

Your process of transformation has taken you through stages of identifying, experiencing, and eventually working through your core issues. You were able to recognize past experiences that influenced your current behaviors and gently and steadily cast off negative influences. You grew stronger in the process, and you probably feel like a survivor. However, being a survivor is not good enough, and you should avoid the word *survivor*. Describing yourself as a survivor is like wearing a badge reminding you and everyone else of your past plight. Moving on to transformation is taking on a new form, a new being. As a new creation, you are whole, healthy, and integrated; you have shed the remnants of your troubled past. You have not just survived. You have overcome!

EXERCISE

List major transformations you have made up to now that show you are overcoming your past.

1. Spiritual:

_____

_____

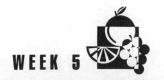

2. Thinking:

_____

_____

3. Emotional:

_____

_____

4. Physical:

_____

_____

PHYSICAL:
Food Cues

Many overeaters feel compelled to eat when food is readily available or visible. A full candy dish in plain view may prove tempting each time you pass by. Try replacing the dish of candy with a bowl of fresh fruit, and perhaps eating the healthier foods will satisfy your food urge. Place your most tempting foods in opaque containers, and keep them stored out of sight.

EXERCISE 1

1. What are trigger foods for you?

_____

2. How will you deal with your trigger foods?

_____

_____

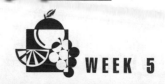 **WEEK 5**

3. What other situations and places trigger munching?

_____

_____

4. What steps will you take to avoid these situations and places?

_____

_____

When Jenny went grocery shopping, she usually walked first by the bakery section. She loved the smell of fresh rolls and pastries. Some days she resisted, but on stressful days she purchased a freshly made cinnamon bun. The cookie and candy aisles also seemed to have loving arms that reached out and grabbed her.

After a grueling day at work, Jenny looked forward to stopping off at a drive-through, telling herself she would just get a cola. Inevitably, she ordered fries or dessert to hold her over until dinner. At times she ordered a jumbo meal because it was easier than preparing dinner. For Jenny, the drive-through became a symbol of relief from the pressure she felt at work.

EXERCISE 2

1. Do you have a favorite bakery, convenience store, or fast-food place you visit daily for a food fix? If so, how can you change your routine to avoid temptation?

_____

_____

2. Think about how you do your shopping. Do you look forward to the cookie, candy, or ice-cream aisles? What aisles do you need to avoid to assist your weight control goal?

_____

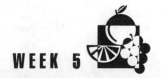

WEEK 5

Is It Worth Saving?

If you are reluctant to throw away leftovers, keeping your goal in mind, try following these suggestions.

Prepare enough food for one average portion per person. Determining the amount needed for each meal will make leftovers unnecessary. (Still, this involves a lot of guesswork, and you will not always guess right.)

If you do have leftovers, immediately place them in opaque containers marked to indicate the leftovers will be used for a specific future meal. You have then committed that food to another meal, placing it off-limits for now.

Unless you are going to eat the leftovers in a day or two, freeze them. Impulsive overeating is less likely when food is frozen.

If possible, assign taking care of leftovers to someone who will not be tempted to overeat. If that is not an option, quickly handle the matter, and move away from the food area.

EXERCISE

1. Do you need to make changes in your view of waste and saving before you can take the steps noted? What are they?

_____

_____

2. What changes can you make so that you and your family learn the amount of food needed to satisfy hunger without overeating?

_____

_____

3. Would you and your family consider having fruits, vegetables, and liquids for seconds instead of the main dish to break the habit of automatic overeating?

_____

_____

 **WEEK 5**

Set Gentle Rules and Abide by Them

If circumstances allow, try to eat at the table as a family. But at times, you and your family may want or need to eat while in the car, in front of a TV, or at other places outside the usually designated eating area. To avoid making the meals eat-until-you're-stuffed events, keep as much structure and routine as possible. For example, give each person a set portion of food, and clear the plates when they determine they are no longer hungry. Then go to the next activity.

Contrast this structured approach to laying out all available food buffet style with open bags of chips, cookies, candy, and so on. The latter encourages open-ended eating, usually well beyond what is needed to satisfy hunger. Using small plastic sandwich bags is an easy way to give each person a portion of food.

As a general rule, agree that the family won't eat while watching TV. Try to break the habit of mindless munching while you are viewing TV, watching movies, or driving.

EXERCISE

What patterns of unhealthy eating practices have you noticed at your family meals? What new methods will you try to ensure appropriate food portions, beginning and ending of eating period?

_____

_____

_____

_____

The Suggestion Box Is Open!

When you eat at fast-food places, try the following suggestions rather than take what is stated on the menu:

- Ask that buns not be grilled in oils or butter.
- Ask for meat to be well done.

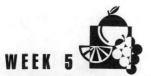

WEEK 5

- Order the smallest portion of fries, chips, or onion rings.
- Get a regular order of fries and divide it instead of ordering each person more fries than needed to satisfy hunger.
- Ask for small containers so that soft drinks and shakes can be split if portions are large.
- Avoid the lure of ordering the largest amount of food and drinks for less money. You might save a few cents, but you will gain unwanted pounds.

These suggestions require that you be assertive in asking for what you want and dealing with those who might question portion amounts. Determine if you need training and practice in this area. (A given is that you always make courteous requests and replies.) Try these suggestions and note the outcome.

Special Touches Are Not Just for Company

Demonstrate to yourself that you are worth a special table setting by using different place mats, nice dishes, lit candles of your favorite color, and soothing background music. Place a flower arrangement in the dining area. Create a relaxing, enjoyable mood for eating.

These extra touches not only remind you to nurture yourself but also signal the beginning and ending of a meal. Instead of nibbling and grazing, make an effort to set a nice table, and use it as a cue that meals begin and end at the table.

When you are relaxed, you are less likely to eat your food quickly before you have a chance to enjoy the meal. Even if your plate is not empty, stop eating when you no longer feel hunger. This seems to be the greatest challenge of the person obsessed with food. Eating only at the table and only for nourishment will reduce the likelihood you will continue to eat or pick at leftovers.

Once you clear the table, enjoy a relaxing cup of tea, and focus on relating to your family. Try this at least two meals per week and then

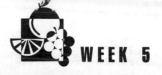

WEEK 5

as often as you can. If you are not in a family situation, do nice things for yourself. You are special, so treat yourself in special ways.

EXERCISE 1

1. What can you do to create an enjoyable eating environment?

_____

_____

2. What makes it difficult for you to do this?

_____

_____

3. List solutions to overcome these difficulties:

_____

_____

EXERCISE 2

1. Where do you usually eat? Check locations where you currently eat food:

___ In bed.

___ In front of the TV.

___ Around the house while doing chores.

___ At the stove while preparing dinner.

___ At the counter while making kids' lunches.

___ In the car while driving.

___ In the kitchen during long telephone conversations.

___ At the mall.

___ On the couch.

___ At the ballpark or the movies.

___ In the car while waiting for kids.

___ Other: _____.

2. Carry a small bottle of water with you and drink instead of eat while shopping. Listen to soothing music when you are in your car. These methods will divert your attention from food. Can you think of other ways to take your mind off food?

_____

_____

Dining Out

According to a report from the National Restaurant Association in the late 1980s, customer pressure caused 73 percent of restaurants to lighten their menus: less meat, less fat, and more fish. Still, more than an average portion of food is served in many restaurants. Assume this is the case. Ask the waiter to bring a "to go" container when your food is served. Immediately place half the food in the container, and put it aside to take with you. Store the food for a later meal, or share it with another. If leftovers are too tempting to be kept, you may need to dispose of them.

Consider the following:

- Ask for smaller portions.
- Order half a sandwich and soup.
- Tell the waiter not to bring certain items, such as fries, chips, or bread.
- Ask to substitute fresh fruits, tomatoes, or low-fat cottage cheese for fries and high-fat salads.
- Order salad dressing on the side.
- Ask for fish baked, broiled, or poached if it's listed as grilled.
- Have the waiter take your plate away as soon as you are no longer hungry, even if food remains.

You are a paying guest, and you deserve what you want. Be polite, but firm. You may not be in a situation to leave if you are met with an uncooperative attitude; however, you do not have to plan a return trip.

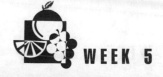

WEEK 5

Crash Course in Menu Language

Descriptive words in menus look and sound delicious—just as they were designed to do. However, if you are weight and health conscious, you would benefit by knowing what you are ordering before the items are served and it is too late to do anything but indulge.

- *Meunière*—rolled in flour and sautéed in butter
- *Fritto*—fried
- *Tempura*—dipped in batter and deep-fried
- *Croquettes*—coated with egg and bread crumbs and deep-fried
- *Béarnaise* and *hollandaise*—rich sauces made with egg yolks and butter
- *Au beurre*—cooked in butter
- *Carbonara*—pasta sauce containing cheese and bacon
- *À la king*—cream sauce
- *Parmigiana*—smothered in cheese

EXERCISE 1

1. Write out sample menus using some or all of the terms above. First, use only the term itself; then, write out the menus using only the definitions.

_____

_____

_____

_____

_____

_____

2. Refer to the menus you have just created. Would you be more likely to order items from the first set of menus or the second?

_____

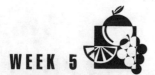

3. To what extent would full description menus alter your food selections, if at all?

_____

_____

_____

EXERCISE 2

Role-play making special requests to restaurant servers. Have a friend play the waiter and act disgusted at times in response to requests being made. Also, practice declining a free basket of chips or bread. Then reverse roles and experience your reaction to such requests. It may take time and practice to make the changes. Be patient and keep practicing.

EXERCISE 3

List foods you will consider giving up or eating less of now. List substitutes you will consider to help you achieve your weight management goal.

Do Away with This:

1. _____
2. _____
3. _____
4. _____

Healthier Substitutes:

1. _____
2. _____
3. _____
4. _____

Food Habits: Time for Changes

EXERCISE 1

1. How often do you eat meals away from home? Record time and place.

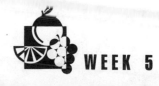

WEEK 5

Breakfast: _____

Lunch: _____

Dinner: _____

2. How do you think your body size affected your life?

_____

3. Think about how you can make healthier choices in your food habits. Are you reluctant to make changes? Why?

_____

EXERCISE 2

1. When and where do you do most of your impulsive eating?

_____

2. What are you feeling while you are eating?

_____

3. How can you structure your day so that you are not interacting with food so much?

_____

4. Check the following changes you will try:

__ Let older siblings prepare lunches and snacks for younger siblings.

__ Prepare next meal when I'm not hungry and freeze/refrigerate it.

__ Keep meals simple and easy to prepare. Use slow cooker (which requires less thought, but produces nice meals).

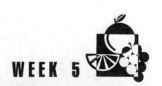

— Keep kids on eating schedule, but not too rigid, so food is accessed only during predictable times.

— Mentally distance myself from food I am preparing and serving.

Asking for Seconds. Many people from our Gentle Eating groups report they struggle resisting food if it is in front of them. Similar to their need to eat everything on their plates is their compulsion to eat as long as food is available in the pots and pans. We suggest that you prepare enough for each family member to have a moderate serving of the main dish. Have fruits and vegetables available if family members still feel hungry. Serving one portion of the main course communicates it should be sufficient.

When you serve food, we suggest that in addition to gauging how much food each person will need, keep all food remaining in the serving dishes off the table. If convenient, clean up, put food away, then eat.

Measuring Progress. Log your setbacks and disappointments as well as your successes on your Progress Chart so you can learn where you need to strengthen your resolve. Note your progress, but recognize that getting off track at times is part of your weight maintenance journey. Expect it and view it as part of the process, not as failure. Learn from your experiences, forgive yourself if you slip, and focus on your goals.

Slow Down Your Eating

1. Eat vegetables and fruits slowly.
2. Stop to take sips of water to enhance fullness and aid digestion.
3. Chew all foods slowly and completely.
4. Eat with your nondominant hand.
5. Focus your attention on conversation with dining companions.
6. Rate your hunger level on the 0–10 scale (with 0 = starved, 5 = satisfied, 10 = stuffed) midway through the meal.

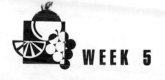

7. Wait five to ten minutes before you finish food on your plate. Reevaluate your hunger level to determine if you wish to continue eating.

8. At the end of the meal, remove all food and dishes promptly.

9. Engage in pleasant conversation as you sip a hot cup of tea or coffee.

EXERCISE

Referring to 6 above, record the experience and outcome of your diversion tactic.

_____

_____

You do not have to respond immediately to your hunger pangs because feelings of hunger come and go. Next time you feel hungry, divert your attention from food for fifteen to thirty minutes—notice how your pangs subside. Learn patience; it is a soothing asset.

Gently Remove Unhealthy Foods

Gradually remove junk food and other foods you tend to overeat. Start by continuing to use foods the family is familiar with; serve smaller portions and slowly introduce alternatives. Do not keep calorie-rich foods handy; place them in opaque containers and make access more difficult.

If you have difficulty managing your eating habits, you may tend to be oversensitive to the behavior and remarks of others. In particular, if you are not in charge of stocking food supplies, you may resent being denied certain foods you found comforting. And if you question the absence of such foods, you may find explanations upsetting. It is unrealistic to think you will never again buy or eat some of your favorite items. So, rather than think of being deprived, consider it a vacation from foods that hinder your weight goal. Make choices that are consistent with reaching your goal of becoming more fit.

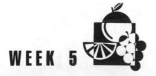

WEEK 5

PROGRESS CHART

Check all that apply.

Spiritual Changes

___ Had at least a fifteen-minute daily quiet time.

___ Memorized a Bible verse.

___ Met with midweek church group.

___ Went to church services.

___ Prayed.

___ Felt a little closer to the Lord.

___ Expressed true feelings to God.

___ Honestly evaluated my relationship with God.

Thinking Changes

___ Recognized and recorded a distorted thought.

___ Experienced change in how I view myself.

___ Experienced change in how I thought about a situation.

___ Was able to develop more accurate/balanced view of person, event, etc.

Emotional Changes

___ Recorded my feelings.

___ Evaluated feelings before eating.

___ Expressed feelings in appropriate manner.

___ Noticed impact a person, place, or event had on my urge to eat.

___ Identified a past trauma or hurt.

___ Sought support from a trusted person.

___ Expressed hurt or pain in appropriate way.

___ Noticed how past hurt was related to urge to eat.

___ Worked on a stage of grief.

___ Noticed a change in level of a negative emotion.

___ Noticed a different reaction to person, place, or event that used to evoke emotional upset.

___ Implemented clear, personal emotional boundaries.

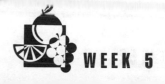

PROGRESS CHART

Check all that apply.

Physical/Behavioral Changes

___ Charted my eating patterns.

___ Did workbook exercises.

___ Tried a new low-fat recipe.

___ Performed at least ten minutes of physical activity.

___ Listened to or watched ten to twenty minutes of a relaxation tape (audio or video).

___ Took at least fifteen minutes for myself.

___ Left some food on my plate.

___ Set a nice table with special touches: flowers, tablecloth, candles; listened to soothing music during mealtime; used special dishes.

___ Went shopping when not hungry.

___ Ate intended portions and stopped.

___ Rated hunger level before and after meals.

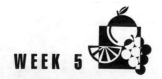

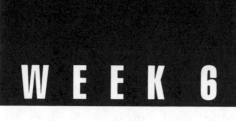

WEEK 6

SPIRITUAL:
Learn to Manage and Express Anger in a Positive Way

■ Jesus referred to the apostles James and John as "Sons of Thunder." The two men were easily angered when they experienced rejection. Over time, through a process of spiritual and behavioral changes, Jesus shaped James and John into men who were quick to love and forgive.

John found he did not have to earn God's love, but it was given freely and abundantly. In turn, John was able to give love freely to others.

Do you have a difficult time controlling your anger? Do you feel anger is a sin and you must repress it? If so, you may be building a reservoir of unresolved feelings, which under stressful conditions can cause you to lose control, hurting yourself and those around you.

You may not reach a stage of rage, but you may act out your anger in more subtle passive ways that can be just as detrimental. Perhaps you feel uncomfortable with this powerful emotion and avoid confrontations that may help resolve your angry feelings. Being unable to be appropriately assertive and express your emotions can lead to feelings of helplessness and low self-esteem. The Bible offers this encouragement: "If you are angry, don't sin by nursing your grudge. Don't let the sun

go down with you still angry—get over it quickly; for when you are angry you give a mighty foothold to the devil" (Eph. 4:26–27 TLB).

When you are upset and repress such feelings, you are susceptible to abusing your mind and body, especially with food. Let God's love and your love of God work together to deal with the harmful feelings and get them behind you.

God implores you, for your sake, for your own good, to deal with your anger promptly. Do not allow unresolved anger to fester in your mind and turn into bitterness and animosity: "Pursue peace with all people, and holiness, without which no one will see the Lord: looking carefully lest anyone fall short of the grace of God; lest any root of bitterness springing up cause trouble, and by this many become defiled" (Heb. 12:14–15).

EXERCISE 1

1. Review the stories of James and John. Note how their relationships with God molded their subsequent behaviors; you might read James 4:7–10 and John 3:4–9, then read others as time permits.

_____

_____

2. How does pent-up distress rob you of spiritual growth, happiness, and joy?

_____

_____

3. There are steps you can take to resolve your feelings. List some of them.

_____

_____

_____

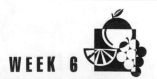

Think of the story of Job and how it teaches you that God can help you deal with your emotions. As time passed, Job grew more and more upset with God, but Job did not deny his feelings of betrayal. He expressed his anger and frustration, he continued to trust God, and eventually, Job's life changed. Expressing his anger was a normal reaction to a series of devastating changes and losses. But Job's patience and faith were rewarded.

It is one of God's promises that if you have unyielding faith and approach Him prayerfully, your prayers will be answered. Jesus said, "If you ask anything in My name, I will do it" (John 14:14).

EXERCISE 2

1. Do you feel that you can express your true feelings about something to God?

_____

Why or why not?

_____

2. Would you tell God you are angry with Him?

_____

3. If you have hostile feelings toward God, have you allowed those feelings to interfere in your relationship with Him?

_____

4. Get your emotions out in the open where you can deal with them; this is an important step toward working through your feelings. List them.

_____

WEEK 6

5. Can you think of appropriate times and places to deal with these strong emotions?

_____

_____

Confrontation? Use Gentle, Firm Assertion!

Again, the story of Daniel provides important lessons you can incorporate into your life. Daniel illustrates how to overcome problems under the most difficult circumstances. He walked the path of the Lord and steadfastly refused to allow any other than God to direct his life.

After being captured and taken from Jerusalem to Babylon, and being installed in the king's household, Daniel and three friends (whose Babylonian names became Shadrach, Meshach, and Abed-Nego) were told by their strong-willed captors to give up the diets they were following and eat only food provided by the king's court. Daniel and his friends questioned the demand for change, for they had firm convictions that they were following God's instructions in their dietary habits. Feeling they could prove their diets were healthier, Daniel and his friends asserted their choices and gained permission to continue their established meals for two weeks. After the allotted time had passed, the youths showed they had more strength and stamina than ones who ate fare served by the court.

Though their actions brought them into conflict with the Babylonians, Daniel and his friends were adamant in following God's revealed will for their lives. And they were vindicated and protected by God from the foreign laws and unstable tyrants they lived under. (Read Dan. 1:5–17.)

Food: A Necessity and Social Focal Point

Food and mealtimes are important in life far beyond required sustenance. In addition to everyday meals, reflect on holidays and special occasions and the role food plays. During both festive and sad times,

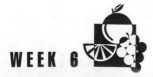

food is and always has been a focal point. Temptation to overeat is especially high when an abundance of food is available and you are experiencing strong emotions such as joy or sadness.

Do Not Let a "Sweet" Situation Turn "Bitter"

For some, the sharing of food, particularly treats, is a deeply felt need. Can you think of someone who provides treats on a regular basis and is offended if you decline to accept a portion? You probably give in, not because you are hungry but because you do not want to hurt feelings. (Never mind that the calorie count is almost equal to the national debt or that it will wreck your dietary habits!) This is not to say the treat is not tempting, but will it be worth the guilt over your momentary loss of resolve?

If you are frustrated over incidents involving proffered food items, in a gentle way let the bearer of such gifts know the efforts are appreciated, but you are trying to lose unwanted pounds. Ask for understanding, and if the person responds with, "Just take a bite or two," be more assertive without being offensive.

Let others know one of your goals is to make wiser choices as you plan, prepare, and eat meals. We hope they will understand and offer low-calorie healthful treats at another time. Regardless, do not fall into the habit of just taking a bite or two. Paul offered these reassuring words: "No temptation has overtaken you except such as is common to man; but God is faithful, who will not allow you to be tempted beyond what you are able, but with the temptation will also make the way of escape, that you may be able to bear it" (1 Cor. 10:13).

EXERCISE

1. List times you gave in and ate treats to keep from hurting feelings. Do you feel that if sugar-laden or fat-rich treats are offered in the future, you will be better able to resist them?

WEEK 6

_____

_____

2. You need to plan meals around ingredients rich in nutritional value but low in calories, emphasizing fruits and vegetables. Visualize yourself in a situation where an abundance of food is offered. Can you pick and choose wisely and bypass foods fried in heavy oils or saturated in rich sauces in favor of foods steamed, baked, or broiled? Search out trays of fresh fruits and vegetables. List several healthful foods you find appealing.

_____

_____

3. Find or create a relaxing atmosphere in which to dine. Make it a fun challenge to turn your dining times into enjoyable experiences, and keep each in your memory bank to enrich your life: "Whether you eat or drink, or whatever you do, do all to the glory of God" (1 Cor. 10:31).

Lord, at times I am unhappy with my life, and I am filled with disappointment. I struggle with problems that I know You will bear if only I turn to You. Help me to avoid all things that will block my progress as I seek to lead a healthy, joyful life. Help me to transfer all my doubts and troubles to the One who has the power to conquer them. Help me to see that when I feel unhappy and disappointed, I am on a darkened pathway, and that is why I stumble and grope about. Light my way, Lord; I seek the many blessings You have promised me. I know that they are mine for the taking if I follow the path You have set for me. Amen.

THINKING:
Body over Mind

With this thinking distortion, you mistakenly assume once food is eaten and in your body, physiological addiction takes place. Therefore,

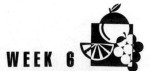

you are powerless to stop and change the outcome during the course of eating. This erroneous thinking often leads to continued overeating and relapse.

Consider the following example: A man started eating a bag of chocolate chip cookies. He assumed since he was addicted to them, he had no control over how many he would eat. Even though he felt bloated and the cookies no longer tasted good, he felt compelled to keep eating. He could have stopped at any point by challenging this distorted belief and saying to himself, "Stop. I can gain control at any time and focus on the future." Instead, negative thinking habits caused this self-talk: "I'm overeating, so I must be unable to stop myself. I may as well not try."

EXERCISE

1. How have you used body over mind rationalizations regarding overeating?

_____

_____

_____

2. What have you learned about continuing or stopping your over-eating behavior?

_____

_____

_____

3. What will you say and do the next time you feel you have no control over your body?

_____

_____

 **WEEK 6**

4. Log in your Thought Record instances when you engage in body over mind distortion.

5. Do you feel you are becoming more adept in identifying and avoiding errors in thinking?

_____

_____

_____

6. Does your mind generate positive responses more readily?

_____

_____

_____

7. Review your previous exercises and focus on all successes you have recorded.

EMOTIONAL:
Transforming Your Life

Your transformation involving spiritual, thinking, emotional, and physical well-being has been described as a train ride. As you move daily toward your goal, ignore the familiar call of "All aboard!" and let the negative STEP off and the positive STEP on. The speed of change is not as important as moving steadily forward. Setbacks and relapses are not moving backward; they are only temporary detours, much like a switch that has been thrown on your track. Learn what causes derailments, devise healthy ways to avoid them, then return to your program. No matter how many switches are thrown (e.g., by people, emotions, circumstances), you can always get back on track! When the climb appears steep, perhaps you can borrow the phrase, "I

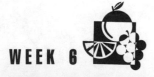

WEEK 6

think I can, I think I can, I think I can," and log in your Progress Chart when your recitation changes to, "I know I can, I know I can, I know I can!"

Peeling an Artichoke

Inner growth and transformation have often been likened to "peeling the layers of an onion." A colleague described it more aptly as "peeling an artichoke." Layer by layer, the false self, the past hurt, and shame are peeled away until you reach the core: the heart.

By the time you complete this workbook, you will have recognized, worked through, and let go of past experiences that have been negatively affecting your adult life. You will become better acquainted with your whole self, and greater joy and peace will fill you as you come to understand who you are in Christ. You will discover your true self: the person you are minus all the negative experiences that have stifled your personal development.

When "No, Thank You" Falls on Deaf Ears

Have you been in a situation where you politely said no to someone offering you food (or more food in the form of seconds or dessert) and the person kept insisting? In the flick of an eye, an otherwise nice individual seemed to make it a mission of the moment to foist food on you and took the matter very personally when you refused.

As you recall the incident, you may be confused by the emotions displayed, which can range from wounded to the core to outright hostility. Probably, you cannot help wondering why it was so important to someone that you chose to eat nothing else. You may never solve that puzzle, just as the one insisting you eat the food may never understand the origin or depth of the emotional reaction to your polite refusal.

To extricate yourself from such incidents, do not take offense at the person's insistence, but do slip into your assertive mode and do not relent in order to appease an unwarranted emotional barrage. There

WEEK 6

are ways to prevent or defuse such confrontations. Some of these ways will be discussed in the following exercises.

EXERCISE 1

1. What feelings did you experience when pressure was applied to change your mind about accepting additional food?

_____

_____

2. What do you usually say in such situations?

_____

_____

3. Which type of person is it most difficult to say "no, thanks" to, especially when the pressuring continues?

_____

_____

4. What have you said or done in the past that made it easier for you to assert yourself regarding food?

_____

_____

EXERCISE 2

Study and review the above questions and your answers, then read the following suggestions for future use:

1. If food is forced on you and you do not want to bring attention to yourself, just take the food. Once others are eating, continue talking, and place the food as far away from you as you can. Be polite and unobtrusive.

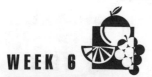

2. You can reply, "I'm full now, maybe later," or "Not now, perhaps later." Either is a good response because you are not making excuses and you are demonstrating to yourself and others present that you respect your body.

3. If a dessert is being offered and your sole reason for declining is that you feel it has too many calories, have alternative desserts in mind or bring your own. (This idea requires that you put your goal and needs ahead of what others may think. Stay focused!)

4. List several scenarios of how you might be pressured and what you might do or say in response. (Be as gentle as possible in your actions and responses, but remain assertive.)

_____

_____

_____

_____

_____

5. Role-play the situations so you can experience your thoughts and emotions. Role-playing also allows you to practice what you will do and say while you cope with your feelings.

EXERCISE 3

1. Which of the suggestions listed above would you likely try?

_____

_____

2. What changes will you have to make first?

_____

_____

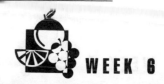

WEEK 6

3. When will you make them?

_____

_____

_____

Lean Back and Learn to Relax

Learn to create a safe place. Get in a comfortable position. Close your eyes, and take a few deep breaths to relax. Imagine a place or activity that creates a feeling of security, calm, and peace within. Perhaps it is a favorite vacation spot or scenery you enjoy. Maybe you are at the beach, lying on the warm sand, or in the mountains, enjoying nature and the cool air.

Let the picture become more defined. Notice what you see there, the sounds, smells, and textures. Link the image you have with one word (Jesus, God, mountains, skiing, beach, warm, cool, etc.). Say the word, repeat the word, see the image, and feel the sensations as you tell yourself to relax. This becomes your safe place. With practice, you can take yourself to your safe place when you feel anxious, fearful, or out of control, or anytime you feel the need to relax. Try going to your safe place when you feel an urge to eat. This will calm you, and you can learn to identify what's fueling the urge; write it down and problem-solve alternative behavior or modes of action other than eating.

EXERCISE

1. My safe place is (describe in detail)

_____

_____

_____

_____

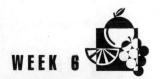

2. I will go there when I feel

_____.

3. I will go there when I feel hurt by

_____.

4. I will go there when I feel stressed or upset by

_____.

Inject Humor as You Deal with Your Food Urges

You probably have never considered that thwarting your food urges could provide fun. Certainly, food urges do not begin on a humorous note according to many of our Gentle Eating group members. They often report an uncontrollable feeling of being pulled by the urge to eat or overeat. After mentally trying to resist the urge, they usually give in, and giving in leaves them feeling powerless and guilty.

The next time you feel a food urge, take a deep breath and relax. Imagine the urge unwinding counterclockwise. You are not going with the urge, blocking, or resisting it; you are dismantling it. Perhaps the urge appears to be unwinding toward you or away from you. Either way, it is demonstrating that you have moment-to-moment power over it. You could imagine the urge transforming into a long, lightly coiled, flexible Slinky, making its way slowly down a long stairway. Watch as gravity allows the Slinky to conquer one step after another, teetering and then continuing downward, end over end, until it reaches the bottom. Watch for a moment as the Slinky sits motionless at the bottom of the stairs. Allow the image to slowly fade. This respite affords you an opportunity to do something else: engage in an activity, or try alternate food or drink more in line with your goal. You can slow down an impulsive, unthinking beeline for food by not acting immediately on your food urge. Using this technique, you can gain time to make

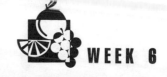

WEEK 6

better decisions. If you consider the food urge beyond your control, it is. If you consider yourself in control, you are.

EXERCISE

1. Following the urge was

_____.

2. My experience with this method was

_____

_____.

3. I noticed the urge increased ___ decreased ___.

As you continue practicing the unwinding/Slinky method, you may find the urge receding and often passing altogether.

Make Up Your Own Message!

Related to the unwinding/transformation method is noticing the food urge and watching it fade. You might see it pass like an airplane pulling a banner past your mind's eye. Do you see a message on the banner, but the letters are too small and you cannot determine what the message is? Direct the airplane to make a wide turn and bring the banner back. This time imagine the letters are even smaller and fainter. Can you read the message by focusing on the banner? You can imagine that the banner passed before you again and you could read the message (make up a humorous one—anything but "Eat at Joe's!"), or you could watch the airplane, with banner trailing, fade from sight.

Do not resist your food urge, and do not reinforce it by turning to food. Use your imagination and make a game of transforming your food urge. Have fun with this! Studies show if you feel the food urge, relax, and just notice it, it likely will fade in intensity and eventually

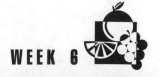

pass. Give your urge an intensity rating, then give it subsequent ratings as it decreases and, perhaps, reappears before it fades altogether. Have an activity or response planned following each urge sequence.

EXERCISE

1. Food urge response:

_____.

2. Intensity rating (0–10 with 0 = starved; 5 = satisfied; and 10 = stuffed):

_____.

3. Overall experience during this exercise:

_____

_____

_____

_____.

Food Urge Got You Down? Lighten Up!

Concentrate on your food urge when it pops up. Rate its intensity, using the 0–10 scale above. If the urge is persistent, instead of attempting to push it aside, allow it to become a momentary star by placing it center stage.

Imagine the food urge as a character, say, a clown. Give it a name. Define its shape and describe its costume: either tall or short, perhaps a baggy polka-dotted suit, long floppy shoes, and large gloved hands. Choose colors for your character and the costume: perhaps a red nose, white circles on cheeks, and fuzzy orange hair.

Continuing the clown theme as an example, choose a setting. Can you see a circus ring? What sounds and smells do you imagine would

WEEK 6

be present? Your imagined sounds could include audience applause, laughter, and vendors calling out, "Balloons! Souvenirs!" Smells might come from hay used to feed circus animals and sawdust covering the circus ring areas. Is the clown under a big top or outdoors? Further describe the surroundings. Is the temperature cool or cold, warm or hot, or just right?

EXERCISE

1. Urge intensity rating (0–10):

_____.

2. Shape:

_____.

3. Color:

_____.

4. The favorite color that I associate with calmness is

_____.

Imagine your favorite calm-colored light is spotlighting the clown/food urge. Concentrate on the stream of light. Allow the light to focus on the clown from every angle as the clown attempts to avoid or dodge the light. Think of the floppy shoes hindering movement. Pretend that an infinite amount of light is available to direct at the clown. Concentrate on the light's path.

You could imagine the heat of the light melting the clown. You could envision the clown hoisting a tiny umbrella overhead, comically trying to elude the light. Now, imagine the clown retreating, shuffling off stage; the stream of light follows, then slowly fades.

Notice what is happening to the food urge throughout the exercise. Is the intensity rating changing?

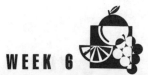

Think of the many scenarios and characters, or shapes, you could choose. Make this exercise a bring-a-smile-to-your-face experiment.

Continue this exercise until you notice a significant change in the urge. When you have finished, take a deep breath and relax.

5. Urge intensity rating (1–10):

_____ .

6. What did you experience during this exercise?

_____

_____

_____

7. This imaging exercise will help when

_____

_____

_____ .

8. This imaging exercise will not help when

_____

_____

_____ .

PHYSICAL:
Listening for Your
Hunger Signals

Infants are born with and listen to their hunger signals. As they develop, they are told what, when, and how much to eat. Gradually, all sense of the feelings of hunger and full is lost. This becomes a foundation for overeating.

WEEK 6

Common practice is to eat until feeling stuffed instead of satisfied. Try to settle on a portion size necessary for you to feel satisfied. Allow your stomach, not your emotions or eyes, to determine when you stop eating.

EXERCISE

Continue to practice rating your hunger level on the scale of 0–10 previously given. Rate the level before, during, after, and fifteen minutes after the meal.

The Myth of Nonfat

Nonfat and low-fat products have inundated the market, but they are not the cure-all answer for the approximately 70 percent of Americans who are still overweight. These products often have the same amount as or more calories than "regular" fat foods. Whether your calories come from fat, protein, or carbohydrates, excess calories convert to fat.

Gentle Eating group members discovered they consumed about twice as much food if it bore a nonfat label. They reported having a compulsion to overeat this "safe" food.

According to a national survey of 2,336 Americans aged eighteen to sixty-five, conducted exclusively for *Parade* magazine by Mark Clements Research and reported in its November 12, 1995, issue, 71 percent of food shoppers are reading food labels, compared with 63 percent in 1991 and 55 percent in 1987. And shoppers remain willing to pay extra for products that are fat-free or contain all-natural ingredients.

The survey found the most popular method for reducing fat is buying low-fat versions of products bought before. Among the respondents who read nutrition labels, 87 percent indicated they paid closest attention to fat content, while 63 percent checked the number of calories from fat.

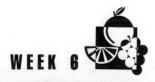

Clearly, Americans are more concerned about their food selections. Being cautious and selective is only the beginning, however. Commitment to lifetime change in lifestyle, involving the four STEPs addressed in this workbook, remains the key to weight management.

EXERCISE

1. Do you put false hope in eating nonfat or low-fat food products?

_____

2. Do you rationalize you can eat or drink more?

_____

3. Do you think a lot about the calories you are saving, then use those "saved" calories to eat more later?

_____

If you answered yes to these questions, perhaps you are choosing foods from technically healthier categories, but you still tend to dwell on food. You may still turn to food when stressed, hurt, angry, or depressed and look in a mirror and lament your shape. You may still weigh yourself before and after you eat, and you may exercise more when you think you have overeaten.

Reviewing your habits concerning weight and referring to your journals and answers to previous exercises will aid you in breaking out of the food deprivation cycle. You *can* do it! Remain focused on your goals.

High Quality Versus Quantity of Food

Filling your body with high-fat, high-sugar foods with few nutrients leaves you feeling unsatisfied. You may enjoy immediate gratification from flavor and texture, but your body still feels hungry and craves healthier foods. Several bingers have told us that after they have gorged on chips, cookies, cake, ice cream, or fries, they feel bloated and uncomfortable, but not nutritionally satisfied. They then eat something healthy to end the craving. Sugar and fat have a place in your daily diet, but not exclusive of high-bulk, high-fiber foods.

EXERCISE 1

1. At your next meal rate your hunger (using the 0–10 scale) before you eat.

_____

2. Tune in to what your body seems to be craving. If it is sugar or fat, rate the urge (0–10). Tell yourself after you eat nutritious food or drink nutritious beverages, you can make another choice if you are still hungry. Eat something healthy that appeals to you. Rate your hunger level while eating. Notice what portion of food it took to reach a level 5 indicating "satisfied." Then rate your hunger level after you finish. Remember to practice leaving some food on your plate. You will learn it takes less food and beverage than you thought to reduce your hunger level.

_____
_____
_____
_____
_____
_____

Several Gentle Eating graduates report not craving junk food or drinks after eating high-quality food and drinking healthy beverages. Of course, you can continue eating and drinking moderate portions

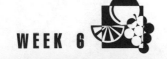

of your favorite junk food and drinks, but try to substitute healthier alternatives.

Do not tell yourself that you *cannot* have certain foods. You may be tempted to rebel by bingeing. Eat nutritious food first, and if you still long for junk food, eat a small portion, select an alternative, or wait until another time.

EXERCISE 2

1. List nutritious food you might enjoy, including vegetables, fruits, whole grains, cereals, and low-fat, high-fiber foods.

_____

_____

_____

_____

2. Search out new items when you food shop and list healthy ones to try.

_____

_____

_____

_____

WEEK 6

PROGRESS CHART

Check all that apply.

Spiritual Changes

___ Had at least a fifteen-minute daily quiet time.

___ Memorized a Bible verse.

___ Met with midweek church group.

___ Went to church services.

___ Prayed.

___ Felt a little closer to the Lord.

___ Expressed true feelings to God.

___ Honestly evaluated my relationship with God.

Thinking Changes

___ Recognized and recorded a distorted thought.

___ Experienced change in how I view myself.

___ Experienced change in how I thought about a situation.

___ Was able to develop more accurate/balanced view of person, event, etc.

Emotional Changes

___ Recorded my feelings.

___ Evaluated feelings before eating.

___ Expressed feelings in appropriate manner.

___ Noticed impact a person, place, or event had on my urge to eat.

___ Identified a past trauma or hurt.

___ Sought support from a trusted person.

___ Expressed hurt or pain in appropriate way.

___ Noticed how past hurt was related to urge to eat.

___ Worked on a stage of grief.

___ Noticed a change in level of a negative emotion.

___ Noticed a different reaction to person, place, or event that used to evoke emotional upset.

___ Implemented clear, personal emotional boundaries.

WEEK 6

PROGRESS CHART

Check all that apply.

Physical/Behavioral Changes

___ Charted my eating patterns.

___ Did workbook exercises.

___ Tried a new low-fat recipe.

___ Performed at least ten minutes of physical activity.

___ Listened to or watched ten to twenty minutes of a relaxation tape (audio or video).

___ Took at least fifteen minutes for myself.

___ Left some food on my plate.

___ Set a nice table with special touches: flowers, tablecloth, candles; listened to soothing music during mealtime; used special dishes.

___ Went shopping when not hungry.

___ Ate intended portions and stopped.

___ Rated hunger level before and after meals.

 **WEEK 6**

WEEK 7

SPIRITUAL:
Acknowledge a Setback
and Make It Temporary

■ Learn to forgive yourself as God forgives you. If you stray from your eating program, view it as a temporary lapse, then get back on track and ask God's help in attaining your goals.

It is counterproductive to indulge in frenzied exercise activities or go on starvation diets. There is no need to self-punish; set realistic goals and work toward them by settling into easy-to-follow, free-of-stress routines. Always keep in mind that you are making a lifetime commitment to God and yourself to pursue a healthful lifestyle. The rewards will include a better self-image, higher self-esteem, and a more responsive mind and body. As you grow spiritually, you will gain more self-control, and the path you have chosen will be an easier one to follow. So if you transgress, forgive yourself immediately and begin anew with renewed resolve!

EXERCISE

1. Think of times you have experienced setbacks in your weight management program. Can you determine if such times are increasing or decreasing in frequency?

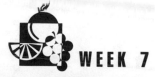

_____

_____

_____

2. Depending on your answer, note the necessary steps to reach your goals. (If such times are increasing, spend more time with God and work on your spiritual growth. If such times are decreasing, take time to thank and praise God for His loving encouragement and support. Note that either answer takes you back to God.)

_____

_____

Is anyone among you suffering? Let him pray. Is anyone cheerful? Let him sing psalms (James 5:13).

Walking and Talking with God

Peter teaches that if you want more and more of God's kindness and peace, you must learn to know Him better and better. Through God's great power, He will provide you with everything you need for living a truly good life.

As you try to do what God wants you to do, He will reveal to you what He wants you to do. You have to put aside your own desires and let God's way prevail.

By following and repeating the steps outlined in the following Scripture, you will grow spiritually and become fruitful and useful to the Lord:

Grace and peace be multiplied to you in the knowledge of God and of Jesus our Lord, as His divine power has given to us all things that pertain to life and godliness, through the knowledge of Him who called us by glory and virtue, by which have been given to us exceedingly great and precious promises, that through these you may be partakers of the divine nature, having escaped the corruption that is in the world through lust. *But also for this very reason, giving all diligence, add to your faith virtue, to virtue knowledge, to knowledge self-control, to self-control perseverance, to perseverance godliness, to godliness brotherly kindness, and to brotherly kindness love. For if these things are yours and abound, you will be neither barren nor unfruitful in the knowledge of our Lord Jesus Christ.* For he who lacks these things is shortsighted, even to blindness, and has forgotten that he was cleansed from his old sins. Therefore, brethren, be even more diligent to make your call and election sure, for if you do these things you will never stumble; for so an entrance will be supplied to you abundantly into the everlasting kingdom of our Lord and Savior Jesus Christ (2 Peter 1:2–11, emphasis added).

EXERCISE

1. Review 2 Peter 1:2–11, and share the good news that you do not have to do things on your own. When you seek to do God's will, you are helped by the power of the Holy Spirit to live a joyful and meaningful life. What can you do today to get to know God and yourself better?

_____

_____

2. Do you realize the importance of keeping your mind and heart focused on God? Note how verses 5–8 (in italics) can be a pattern for your spiritual growth, allowing your life to be enriched daily.

_____

_____

3. How does 2 Peter 1:2–11 show you the way to self-control and better eating habits?

_____

_____

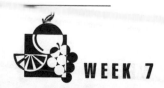

WEEK 7

Lord, again I humbly kneel in prayer to give thanks for Your strength and presence in my life. The loneliness and confusion I felt have been swept away by Your love and power and strength. I partake freely of Your love and power and strength, knowing the source is never ending. Help me to become all that You would have me be: healthy in spirit, healthy in mind, and healthy in body. Walk with me and guide me, I pray. Amen.

THINKING:
Treat Yourself Kindly in Your Head

Over the past six weeks you have been listening to, recording, and changing your self-talk and negative thinking. By now, you are treating yourself more kindly in your head. Differences in your thinking and feelings will become more apparent, and your eating behavior will continue to improve as you learn how to avoid negative thoughts and words that fuel unhealthy eating habits. Positive and encouraging self-talk raises your self-esteem and produces heightened feelings of self-worth.

EXERCISE 1

Read the thinking distortions listed below, and check off ones that apply to you:

__ All or none thinking __ Labeling

__ Overgeneralization __ Personalizing blame

__ Mental filter/selective abstraction __ Catastrophizing

__ Emotional reasoning __ Body over mind

__ "Should" and "shouldn't" statements

EXERCISE 2

1. Read each of the negative thoughts listed below. Indicate by writing 0-10, with 0 = not at all; 5 = somewhat; 10 = totally, the degree you feel each applies to you, if at all.

Negative Thoughts	
___ I can't.	___ I am stupid.
___ I don't deserve to be loved.	___ I am insignificant/unimportant.
___ I am a bad person.	___ I am a disappointment.
___ I am horrible.	___ I deserve to die.
___ I am worthless.	___ I deserve to be miserable.
___ I am shameful sometimes.	___ I cannot get what I want.
___ I am not lovable.	___ I am a failure.
___ I am not good enough.	___ I have to be perfect.
___ I deserve the worst.	___ I should please everyone.
___ I cannot be trusted.	___ I am permanently damaged.
___ I cannot trust myself.	___ I am ugly.
___ I cannot trust my judgment.	___ I should have done something.
___ I cannot succeed.	___ I cannot stand it.
___ I am not in control.	___ I cannot trust anyone.
___ I am powerless.	___ I do not deserve _____.
___ I am weak.	___ I'm invisible.
___ I cannot protect myself.	___ I mustn't make others feel bad.

2. Read each of the positive thoughts in the following list. Indicate by writing 0-10, as previously explained, the degree you feel each applies to you, if at all.

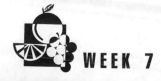

Positive Thoughts	
__ I am a good person.	__ I have done the best I could.
__ I am constantly striving to change for the better.	__ I deserve to live.
__ I have worth.	__ I deserve to be content and happy.
__ I do not deserve to feel shameful.	__ I can get/ask for what I want.
__ I am lovable.	__ I fail/have failed sometimes.
__ I deserve to be loved.	__ Mistakes are okay; I can learn from my mistakes.
__ I am okay as I am.	__ I can do what I need to do.
__ I deserve good things.	__ I am becoming healthy.
__ I can be trusted.	__ I have attractive attributes.
__ I can trust myself.	__ I did what I could at the time.
__ I can trust my judgment.	__ I learned/can learn from it.
__ I can try/learn to.	__ It's over; that was then; I am safe now.
__ I can succeed.	__ I can learn to cope with it.
__ I can be in control.	__ I can choose whom to trust.
__ I have power.	__ I can let it out and let it go with safe people.
__ I am strong.	__ I can have/deserve _____
__ I can establish healthy boundaries.	_____.
__ I can think intelligently.	
__ I am significant/important.	__ I can be seen.

EXERCISE 3

1. Note which positive thoughts you were able to endorse over a level of 4.

_____

_____

_____

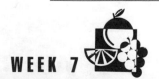

WEEK 7

2. What steps do you have to work on to internalize and believe at a level of 10?

_____

_____

_____

3. What needs to happen before you can believe all the positive statements?

_____

_____

_____

4. What past experiences make it difficult for you to endorse all the positive statements and believe the best about yourself?

_____

_____

_____

EMOTIONAL:
Body Image

Looking in a mirror can become an obsession and is often a trigger for overeating. Do you look in a mirror and focus on what you do not like about your body? Do you tend to overlook your positive qualities and search for negative features? For example, when Jane walks past the mirror, she sees her "fat stomach." Her self-talk is usually, "My stomach looks huge! I can't get the weight off no matter how hard I try. That's it! I'm not eating lunch or dinner today." Jane skips lunch, starts to feel hunger, and becomes preoccupied with food. But the thought of eating something makes her feel anxious because she doesn't want her stomach to stay "fat." By midafternoon, her feelings of hunger

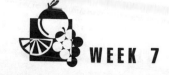

have escalated, and she starts to think about how good a cheeseburger would taste. By the time she drives through her favorite fast-food place she thinks, *Oh, forget it. If I'm going to eat a cheeseburger, I might as well get the big value pack. I'll skip breakfast tomorrow.* So, now she is dealing with a cheeseburger, large fries, and a drink. Later, Jane walks by a mirror and focuses only on her stomach, and the process is repeated.

Concentrating only on what you consider to be your worst features is a form of selective abstraction. Like other negative thinking, it can ultimately lead to overeating. In the exercises below, evaluate how you feel about your body. Notice your self-thoughts and how they might relate to your body image and your eating behavior.

EXERCISE 1

1. If I could, I would make the following changes in my body:

_____

_____

_____.

2. My upper body is

_____.

3. My midsection is

_____.

4. My lower body is

_____.

EXERCISE 2

1. What did your parents or caregivers, siblings, and friends say about your appearance as you were growing up?

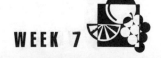

Negative comments: _____

_____.

Positive comments: _____

_____.

2. How did these comments make you feel (e.g., secure, pleased, confident, hurt, mad, angry, sad, rebellious)?

_____

3. What did you say/do in response to these comments?

_____

4. How did these comments influence your body image, view of food, and self-esteem?

_____

_____

Creating a Positive Body Image

EXERCISE 1

1. Keep a body image journal and record the a-b-c chain of negative body image experiences. (a) Antecedents—events and situations that trigger negative thoughts, beliefs, and feelings about your body (for example, while at the beach, at a picnic, in a swimsuit). (b) Beliefs—thoughts about yourself and your body (for example, "My upper arms and stomach are huge!"). (c) Consequences—effect of the event on your feelings and behavior (for example, you feel depressed; you take out a bag of chips and start eating them).

2. Identify any distortions or exaggerations in your view of yourself or the situation. (How likely is it that "everyone" is looking at your

WEEK 7

arms or stomach? Are your thighs really "gross" or simply not toned?) What positive personal traits or abilities do you project, unrelated to physical appearance? Focus on realistic facts.

_____

_____

_____

_____

3. Write down a more objective view of yourself, your body, and the situation. ("I'm not a fat slob, but I do need to lose fifteen or twenty pounds. I am more than my physical appearance.") During this step, think like a detective and look for hard "evidence" for or against the thoughts and beliefs you generated. What did people actually say? How did they actually behave toward you?

_____

_____

_____

_____

4. For relapse prevention, think about a typical situation where the a-b-c sequence occurs. Practice refuting the negative thoughts, focusing on objective evidence (for example, "I'm not a lazy pig; I'm a good mother and competent coworker; I'm very giving"). Identify resistant thoughts, beliefs, or feelings that interfere with your ability to change your body image (for example, "What does it matter what I accomplish if I'm fat?" or "How can I see anything positive about my fat body?"). Negative, distorted views of yourself can trigger an overeating episode. Learn to challenge and change your negative, distorted views.

_____

_____

_____

_____

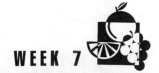

EXERCISE 2

Check which of the following positive changes you will try. Describe the effect of these experiences on your eating behavior.

___ 1. Make a list of your physical attributes that you like (think about compliments or positive evaluations others have made).

_____

___ 2. Reduce the number of times you look into a mirror. This is necessary to break the obsessive negative chain of thinking and behaving. Ultimately, try to look into a mirror only once or twice a day.

_____

___ 3. Refrain from asking others, "Can you tell I've lost weight?"

_____

___ 4. Be gentle with yourself. These are difficult habits to break. Start out slowly and be patient with your setbacks. Negative habits will dissolve if not reinforced.

_____

___ 5. Accept compliments. Period! If you are complimented on articles of clothing you are wearing, do not dilute the comment with, "Yeah, it's the only thing I can fit into!" Just say, "Thank you." Period! Practice this response in advance several times.

_____

___ 6. Resist the common habit of comparing your life (e.g., appearance, eating habits, physical activity) with the lives of others. Changes in this area may be facilitated by recording your comparison patterns. Start by focusing on other people's hair, smiles, eyes, and positive aspects of their nature, not body size, eating habits, and so on. Avoid verbal

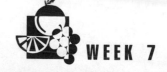

WEEK 7

or self-talk, such as, "Her hair looks so healthy and glossy; mine is always limp and dull"; "He has the nicest smile; I could have a nice smile, too, if my teeth weren't crooked"; "Her eyes look so great, even though she's wearing glasses; my eyes are too close together and my eyebrows are too thin"; "He is so outgoing and popular; if I had nicer clothes and didn't weigh so much, I could be more outgoing and popular."

___ 7. Objectively evaluate whether thin or fit people are actually happier, more successful, and have fewer problems. Chronic dieters often exaggerate how getting thin will change or has changed their lives. Remember, the goal is to be objective—not to say things just to feel better. Look for evidence; try to view the situation in a different way.

___ 8. If you are having a difficult time with obsessive negative thinking, really exaggerate the catastrophic belief: "I'll never stop overeating. I'm going to gain three hundred pounds, be bedridden, and lose all my friends and family." Try to make the supposed outcome horrible. Sometimes this technique helps you to see how distorted your thinking is.

Self-Image

How do you see yourself? Do you view yourself one way when you are with certain people and have a different view when you are with others? Are you engaging in mind reading and projecting what you think others see when they look at you? Practice putting your best foot forward, then evaluate the whole you and not just your appearance.

EXERCISE

1. Write in the degree (0–10 with 0 = not at all; 5 = somewhat; 10 = totally) of the following characteristics you feel best describe you:

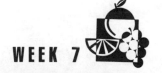

WEEK 7

__ Outgoing	__ Reserved
__ Giver	__ Taker
__ Responsible	__ Irresponsible
__ Leader	__ Follower
__ Confident	__ Not confident
__ Warm	__ Cold
__ Close	__ Distant
__ Brave	__ Afraid
__ Risk taker	__ Risk avoider
__ Smart	__ Dull
__ Good	__ Bad

2. What negative messages from significant adults in your childhood might have influenced your self-image?

_____

_____

3. How does your current self-image relate to your relationship with food?

_____

_____

4. Characteristics from the above list I am pleased to have:

_____

_____

5. Characteristics I feel I need to change:

_____

_____

6. Characteristics I would like to have:

_____

_____

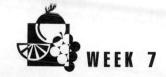

WEEK 7

7. What steps can you take to cast aside undesirable qualities and develop desired qualities?

_____

_____

_____

8. Which of these characteristics did your parents or caregivers say you had as a child or teen?

_____

_____

9. Which of these characteristics did your friends say you had as a child or teen?

_____

_____

10. Using the above list, how do family, friends, and others who are currently in your life describe you now?

_____

_____

_____

_____

PHYSICAL:
Creative Meals Can Be
Easy—Plan Ahead!

You may admire someone who has the ability to prepare pleasing meals in minutes, but think the person has a talent you do not possess. With minimum planning and organizing you can climb to the top of the creative ladder.

Daily meals must be balanced to provide nutrients your body needs to develop, maintain growth, resist infection, and revitalize. To keep mealtimes from being boring and time consuming, take advantage of the many tips and recipes available and suit them to your needs. With few changes, you can make tasty, satisfying dishes containing less fat, less salt, and less sugar. If you have been clinging to calorie-laden recipes, start thinking of substitutions to turn your favorite dishes into healthy choices.

To point you in the right direction, consider the following examples. A savings of 63 calories, 8 grams of fat, and 29 milligrams of cholesterol can be achieved by substituting 8 ounces of skim milk for 8 ounces of whole milk: 8 ounces of whole milk contains 149 calories, 8 grams of fat, and 34 milligrams of cholesterol; 8 ounces of skim milk contains 86 calories, trace amounts of fat, and 5 milligrams of cholesterol.

A savings of 182 calories, 24 grams of fat, and 48 milligrams of cholesterol can be achieved by substituting ½ cup of nonfat yogurt for ½ cup of sour cream: ½ cup of sour cream contains 246 calories, 24 grams of fat, and 51 milligrams of cholesterol; ½ cup of nonfat yogurt contains 64 calories, trace amounts of fat, and 3 milligrams of cholesterol.

First, get organized. Preparing a weekly menu, with one visit to the market for all ingredients, saves time, money, and energy. Plan a fun shopping day. Take lists of needed items and enjoy the movement, sounds, scents, and displays that are the pulse of the store. Have a light snack before you shop to avoid being overly hungry or tempted. Always give a prayer of thanks for the many selections of foods available to nourish your body and for the finances to purchase them.

If you shop with small children, this is a special time to share with them. Answer their questions and encourage their curiosity. The produce department is a wonderful classroom. Teach children to count, recognize colors, name fruits and vegetables, and help you make choices. Manners, math, and money exchange can be intriguing at the checkout stand. However, do not slow the progress of other shoppers.

WEEK 7

Produce/Herbs

Be selective in the produce section. Usually, the best buys are items in season and abundant. Experiment with small amounts of items you have never tried. Some could become new favorites.

Fresh herbs can add intriguing tastes to soups, salads, or main dishes and can be used as garnish. Try basil, bay leaves, cilantro, mint, oregano, parsley, sage, and thyme. Dried herbs are a good backup to keep handy in your pantry.

According to *The New Statistical Abstract of the United States,* published in October 1995, 8 percent of households maintain herb gardens. Creative cooks will surely increase that percentage as they discover new flavors and learn more about health benefits attributable to herbs.

In most supermarkets, there are wide selections of fruits. Fresh orange, lemon, and lime juice will add zip to sauces and salad dressings. Fruit juices can replace milk in some recipes or on cereal. Try small amounts initially; the tastes may not appeal to everyone.

Herbal or fruit-flavored vinegar makes salad dressings and recipes taste treats.

Prepare Produce for Serving and Refrigeration

Rinse greens and herbs, spin dry or pat dry with paper towels, and place in plastic vegetable storage bags.

Rinse and cut celery ribs, carrots, radishes, green onions, broccoli, and cauliflower into bite-sized pieces. Drain on paper towels, then store in individual plastic vegetable bags or plastic containers with lids for cooking, snacks, or salads. An assortment can be arranged on a dish for snacks after school or after work and is great for "on the road" munching.

Save parings from vegetables for soup stock. Place in a pan, cover with water, season, cook, strain, store or freeze. Bouillon cubes will add more flavor. "A soup appetizer may help you diet," says Henry A. Jordan, M.D., who analyzed 100,000 meals of 500 volunteers at

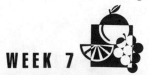

the University of Pennsylvania's Wharton Center for Applied Research. "Nearly a hundred calories less per meal were eaten when soup was an appetizer."

Buy cut melons for smaller quantities and more variety. Peel, slice, cube or ball, and store in plastic containers with lids for quick serving.

Puree cooked fresh vegetables in a blender or food processor to substitute for butter, milk, or cream when making creamed soups.

Pureed vegetables can be frozen in ice cube trays to defrost as needed; they are especially useful to feed infants and small children.

Prepare Meat, Fish, and Fowl for Refrigeration or Freezing

Remove all items from original wrappings and rinse thoroughly. Divide into individual portions and wrap. Place one serving for each family member into a large freezer bag. This speeds defrosting and meal preparation.

Boil cleaned and dressed fowl in water seasoned with onion, garlic, celery, and green pepper. Strain and use broth (instead of fat or oil) to stir fry or coat pasta (cooked and drained) before adding sauce. When cooking rice, use broth in place of water for added flavor.

Remove all bones and fat from meat purchases. Dispose of fat, freeze bones in freezer bag, label, and date. To use, boil in water seasoned with onion, garlic, celery, cilantro, green pepper, dry onion soup mix, and stewed tomatoes for a soup base. (Discard bones after you have prepared soup base.)

For useful and important information on handling and storing meat and poultry, plus much more, you can call the United States Department of Agriculture's hotline at this toll-free telephone number: 1-800-535-4555. Specialists are available to assist you Monday through Friday from 10:00 A.M. to 4:00 P.M., eastern standard time.

Salads

Fresh raw vegetables contain a wealth of vitamins and minerals that refresh and energize you. Varied combinations of fruits, vegetables,

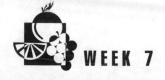

WEEK 7

seafood, chicken, dairy products, and meats can be made into salads with unique tastes, colors, textures, and shapes. Consider the importance of visual appeal when preparing meals. You may want to arrange individual vegetables, greens, other selections, and salad dressings on a table or buffet for each family member to put together a salad. This serving method saves money by eliminating waste and gives family members a choice.

To create a creamy dressing or vegetable dip, use plain yogurt as a base and add fresh herbs such as coriander or parsley with a touch of lime juice. For a tangy variation, add dill, curry powder, or horseradish.

Balsamic vinegar has a deeper, sweeter taste than cider varieties. Use sparingly on strong-flavored greens such as watercress, arugula, or radicchio. For a tangy-tasting low-fat dressing, combine with fresh lemon or lime juice on romaine or delicate greens, or mix with a little Dijon mustard.

Potatoes, Rice, and Pasta

These foods, usually classified as fattening, are often avoided by weight watchers. However, it is not the foods, but what you put on or mix with them, that earn them this label. Potatoes, rice, and pasta contain valuable nutrients, are versatile in presentation, are always available, and are inexpensive. These foods should be cooked thoroughly, and they may be flavored with onions, garlic, herbs, spices, or light sauces. Serve as a side dish or main entree.

Nonfat yogurt may replace sour cream in many recipes and is especially good on baked potatoes.

Pastry

For quick preparation of quiches, strudels, pies, spring rolls, and pizza, buy refrigerated or frozen dough, puff pastry, and pizza bases. Check ingredients, and avoid products containing additives or animal fats. You can prepare bake-ahead dishes on a weekend and freeze them, saving meal preparation time during a busy week.

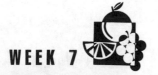

WEEK 7

Mexican Dishes

Tacos, enchiladas, burritos, and nachos are nutritious, give your menus variety, and are inexpensive. Here are some ways to reduce fat:

- Heat tortillas or tortilla chips in microwave or oven. Do not fry.
- Stir-fry vegetables in vegetable stock or nonfat chicken broth.
- Use vegetarian beans (do not refry), baked and shredded chicken or roast, and nonfat cheese.
- Bake chicken or roast in a plastic cooking bag. Chicken and roast can be baked, shredded, and frozen ahead of time and used in other recipes.
- Finely chop lettuce, onions, tomatoes, and cilantro.
- Finely grate nonfat cheese.
- Place all ingredients on a table or buffet in separate containers for family members to make their own.
- Serve with side dishes of rice, salad, and fruit in season.

Desserts

Desserts are a pleasure almost everyone enjoys, and there is no need to delete them from your meals. The key to eating desserts is the same as for all other foods: eat in moderation and limit amounts of fat and sugar.

Fresh fruits and berries are always good dessert choices. Buy in quantity when they are in season. Berries can be rinsed and frozen as they are, and many fruits can be rinsed, pared, and frozen; however, rinse, pare, cook, and puree apples to freeze. You can use a variety of toppings to make beautiful, healthy desserts.

Experiment with flavors and substitute ingredients to achieve healthy menus you and your family will enjoy. Get creative! Mealtimes can be a true treat: good, healthy food, well prepared, for taste; pleasing presentation, for visual appeal; nice surroundings and soothing sounds, for an enjoyable occasion.

WEEK 7

PROGRESS CHART

Check all that apply.

Spiritual Changes

__ Had at least a fifteen-minute daily quiet time.

__ Memorized a Bible verse.

__ Met with midweek church group.

__ Went to church services.

__ Prayed.

__ Felt a little closer to the Lord.

__ Expressed true feelings to God.

__ Honestly evaluated my relationship with God.

Thinking Changes

__ Recognized and recorded a distorted thought.

__ Experienced change in how I view myself.

__ Experienced change in how I thought about a situation.

__ Was able to develop more accurate/balanced view of person, event, etc.

Emotional Changes

__ Recorded my feelings.

__ Evaluated feelings before eating.

__ Expressed feelings in appropriate manner.

__ Noticed impact a person, place, or event had on my urge to eat.

__ Identified a past trauma or hurt.

__ Sought support from a trusted person.

__ Expressed hurt or pain in appropriate way.

__ Noticed how past hurt was related to urge to eat.

__ Worked on a stage of grief.

__ Noticed a change in level of a negative emotion.

__ Noticed a different reaction to person, place, or event that used to evoke emotional upset.

__ Implemented clear, personal emotional boundaries.

PROGRESS CHART

Check all that apply.

Physical/Behavioral Changes

___ Charted my eating patterns.

___ Did workbook exercises.

___ Tried a new low-fat recipe.

___ Performed at least ten minutes of physical activity.

___ Listened to or watched ten to twenty minutes of a relaxation tape (audio or video).

___ Took at least fifteen minutes for myself.

___ Left some food on my plate.

___ Set a nice table with special touches: flowers, tablecloth, candles; listened to soothing music during mealtime; used special dishes.

___ Went shopping when not hungry.

___ Ate intended portions and stopped.

___ Rated hunger level before and after meals.

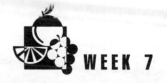

WEEK 7

SPIRITUAL:
Relapse? Regroup!

■ God understands you and your needs. Study His Word, and it will provide guidelines to help you prepare for, avoid, and recover from setbacks you may experience.

If you feel your resolve weakening and you are suffering relapses, regroup and prayerfully call upon God for strength. Do not allow feelings of despair and hopelessness to set in, making you wonder if continuing your program is useless. Let God know you have faith in Him and rely on His power. Gently admonish yourself that there is no need to wait until these feelings loom like large, dark clouds in your mind before you turn to God. Remind yourself that your God is a God of new beginnings: "Then He who sat on the throne said, 'Behold, I make all things new.' And He said to me, 'Write, for these words are true and faithful'" (Rev. 21:5).

God is patient with you, and you must be patient with yourself. You are not on a solitary journey; God is always with you. Associate with others who are traveling the path you have chosen, and think of ways in which you can help and encourage each other. Shared experiences can be enjoyable and rewarding. Remember your past mistakes just long enough to know they caused you to stray from your path, then forget them and move forward: "Return, you backsliding children, and I will heal your backslidings" (Jer. 3:22).

EXERCISE

1. Read Amos 9:11–15 to learn more about new beginnings. Reflect on this truth: God's loving forgiveness is everlasting; setbacks are only temporary. Note your thoughts.

_____

_____

_____

2. Search out and list other Scriptures that speak to you about setbacks and how to avoid or overcome them.

_____

_____

_____

Give Up "Me-Centered" for "Christ-Centered"

You are changed from within by experiencing the love of God. By studying Luke, you learn that the Holy Spirit inundates your heart with God's love. As you experience and understand God's love, you will strive to stay in fellowship with Him. You will follow His directions to make significant changes in your character and learn the importance of loving God and others as God instructed you to do. Recall that He said this was His supreme commandment to you.

Treat others as you want them to treat you. Do you think you deserve credit for merely loving those who love you? Even the godless do that! And if you do good only to those who do you good—is that so wonderful? Even sinners do that much! And if you lend money only to those who can repay you, what good is that? Even the most wicked will lend to their own kind for full return! Love your enemies! Do good to them! Lend to them! And don't be concerned about the fact that they won't repay. Then your reward from heaven will be very great, and you will truly be acting as sons of God: for he is kind to

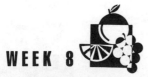

WEEK 8

the unthankful and to those who are very wicked. Try to show as much compassion as your Father does. Never criticize or condemn—or it will all come back on you. Go easy on others; then they will do the same for you. For if you give, you will get! Your gift will return to you in full and overflowing measure, pressed down, shaken together to make room for more, and running over. Whatever measure you use to give—large or small—will be used to measure what is given back to you (Luke 6:31–38 TLB).

You will see how everything in life falls into place when you walk and talk with the Lord and give Him power over your life. Being associated with others in Christian fellowship and being accountable to other believers are vital to living a life that is Christ-centered: "Beloved, I pray that you may prosper in all things and be in health, just as your soul prospers" (3 John 2).

EXERCISE

1. Read and list several promises God makes to you in His Word.

_____

_____

_____

2. List ways you can give up your me-centered life as you seek a Christ-centered life.

_____

_____

_____

3. Make Christ a daily part of your life. List times you might set aside to be in fellowship with other believers to strengthen your faith and increase your knowledge of God and His promises to you. (Make

225

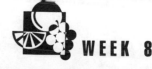

WEEK 8

these times of fellowship and learning looked-forward-to events, and enter into them with enthusiasm!)

_____

_____

_____

All Work and No Play . . .

Taking time for fun and leisure is essential in maintaining balance and overall good health. Finding time is most often the problem. Jesus needed and took time to re-create, relax, rest, and be alone: "There remains therefore a rest for the people of God. For he who has entered His rest has himself also ceased from his works as God did from His" (Heb. 4:9–10).

Find ways to meet your need for these important pursuits and reduce stress in your life.

EXERCISE

1. Think of some fun activities you wish you could do.

_____

_____

_____

_____

2. Can you find time for at least one enjoyable, fun activity this week? What activity would you schedule if you could?

_____

_____

3. What would you have to give up to set aside time for yourself?

_____

_____

_____

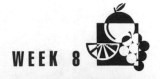

4. Would this cause problems in your life?

_____

_____

5. If you cannot set aside the time you feel is necessary all at once, can you take mini-breaks?

_____

_____

6. Paul reminds you that being spiritually fit is more important than being physically fit. Paul told Timothy to "spend [his] time and energy in the exercise of keeping spiritually fit" (1 Tim. 4:7 TLB). Paul was referring to a daily discipline of spiritual development. Combine your talks with God with walks with God, and the results will change you in body as well as spirit. Describe some of the changes.

_____

_____

> Therefore my heart is glad, and my glory rejoices;
> My flesh also will rest in hope (Ps. 16:9).

7. List some changes you will consider to develop a firm foundation of faith in the Lord. Always take a gentle approach toward your dietary and exercise habits.

_____

_____

As you therefore have received Christ Jesus the Lord, so walk in Him (Col. 2:6).

Lord, You have wrought many wonderful changes in my life. I recognize and feel the need to tell others of the comfort and strength You have given me. Help me to be a powerful voice to spread Your Word. Let me radiate the joy You have brought to me, and let others

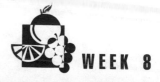

WEEK 8

be drawn to the warmth so that they will want to seek the Source. Help me to find the right time and the right place and the right words to convey to others the magnificent possibilities that You will bring to them if only they acknowledge and believe. I pray that others see in me a new person—healthier, happier, and more content—and that You make of me a shining example. Amen.

THINKING:
Sidetracked? Not for Long!

When you generally follow your weight management program, you feel a sense of personal control. This feeling of control usually lasts until you face a high-risk situation such as an emotional upset or a party with tables and trays of tempting food available; then negative thinking may cause you to slip or deviate from your plan.

For example, you may make negative self-statements, such as, "Oh, no, not chocolate cake! I won't be able to handle this." Or you may focus more on the positive aspects of the food, such as, "This will taste so good; it will help me relax." Positive fantasies regarding food tend to be remembered more than the negative effects of overeating (e.g., abdominal pain, weight gain). So, to help you through some high-risk situations, you may have to make friends with moderation rather than abstinence.

To reduce conflict between how you see yourself ("I can stay on my program") and your behavior ("I am overeating"), you may try to adapt your thinking to accommodate the situation and continue to overeat. The dialogue becomes: "What's the use? I really can't control my eating, so I might as well just keep eating." Feeling helpless and at times hopeless about your ability to change, you continue overeating, reinforcing your view of yourself as an overeater. Then you attribute your behavior to a lack of willpower or personal shortcomings, "I don't have what it takes," rather than to poor coping strategies, which can be changed.

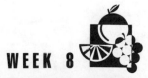

Relapse Prevention: Remember I CAN!

*I*dentify high-risk situations.

*C*oping skills—learn methods to avoid or overcome high-risk situations.

*A*ctual high-risk situations allow practice time for coping skills.

*N*ote positive successes—review for encouragement.

Keep a Relapse Log

Use the following questions to keep a journal of lapses, indicating when, where, with whom, and why you think the lapse took place. Notice any patterns and develop strategies to cope with such situations.

1. Describe the lapse:

_____.

2. Location (home, work, car, restaurant, etc.):

_____.

3. Other people present:

_____.

4. What was happening? (What was going on? What was said? Any triggers?)

_____

5. What were you feeling?

_____

6. What thoughts (distorted beliefs) preceded the feeling?

_____

7. What did you do?

_____

8. What can you do differently next time? (Take time to practice and imagine your new responses, thinking, and behavior.)

Describe Your Relapse Fantasy

In your mind, go over the specifics of a possible relapse in a setting of your choice. What will happen? Why does it happen? What will you do? Visualize yourself effectively handling the situation, and experience the feeling of satisfaction you gain.

Practice until you feel comfortable with the coping methods you have settled on. Now go out in the real world and gently, but decisively, turn the fantasy into reality. (Remember: I CAN!)

EMOTIONAL:
Make Sure Unfinished
Business Is Your Own

Parents or caregivers often have remnants of past unresolved issues that, knowingly or unknowingly, can be passed on to children. Parents or caregivers may want children to achieve or accomplish what the parents or caregivers have not (e.g., college, career, financial security, sports, popularity). These predetermined expectations can hinder children in achieving their potential and are a frequent source of conflict among family members.

EXERCISE 1

Review the following list and try to determine whether you knowingly or unknowingly heap your unresolved issues and aspirations on your children:

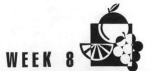

1. Do you have a career you like?

_____

2. Do you consider yourself to be financially successful?

_____

3. Do you have any goals you have not met? If so, what are they?

_____

4. Do you feel capable of reaching those goals?

_____

5. Do you feel successful in your career?

_____

6. What is your usual emotional relationship with authority figures (e.g., bosses, police, teachers)?

_____

7. How comfortable do you feel about your sexuality?

_____

8. How comfortable do you feel about your body?

_____

9. What fears do you still have (e.g., shyness, taking risks, fear of failure)?

_____

10. List any areas you feel your children are working out for you.

_____

_____

WEEK 8

11. Can you think of ways to resolve these issues so your children do not have to stand in for you?

EXERCISE 2

1. What issues or unresolved desires do you feel your parents or caregivers "dumped" or "wished" on you?

---

2. What unrealistic roles or standards do you want to give back to your parents or caregivers?

---

3. What negative feelings or emotions (e.g., pain, anger, hurt, fears) would you like to give back to your parents or caregivers?

EXERCISE 3

Reflect on how your life might have been different without the pressure or presence of your parents' or caregivers' agenda. Relax, take several comfortable breaths, and when you are ready, close your eyes and imagine a large black bag. Imagine putting all of the emotional baggage your parents or caregivers heaped on you into that black bag. One by one, put in guilt, shame, high expectations, disappointments. When you are finished, close the bag. Now, imagine handing the bag over to your parents or caregivers. Everything you want to return is there in that black bag: all the negative comments, all the things they have inadvertently said and done that have limited your growth. After you have handed over the bag, notice how free you feel. Do you feel that a great pressure has been lifted from you? Walk away and enjoy the feeling.

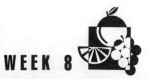

1. What did you put into the black bag?

_____

2. What do you feel unsure about? Are there things you are hesitant to release? Why?

_____

Make a decision today to let go of all past influences that have inhibited your ability to see yourself as God sees you. Then you will be free to reach your full potential.

Marriage, Food, and Weight

Perhaps your weight management problems began after your marriage. If you determine there is a connection regarding your food, body, and weight management issues, what would you like your spouse to do differently? Rate the quality of your marriage. Use realistic guidelines, such as common interests, mutual respect, feelings of love and kindness, helpfulness, supportiveness, and so on. Determine if some areas indicate a need for change. Do you feel at ease in communicating with your spouse, or do you dread verbal encounters involving issues on which you differ? Finding healthy ways to relate to your spouse, to negotiate, and to solve your problems may reduce your dependency on food as a tool to cope.

A Gentle Eating group member shared her story. Joan and her husband had been married five years. Her husband received a promotion, which required relocation. Joan had recently completed graduate school and was offered what she considered a once-in-a-lifetime opportunity where they currently resided. Though she wanted her husband to continue his climb toward greater success, she felt she could not deny herself the career offer. She did not feel she could completely place her faith in God to find her a good opportunity if she moved to the new location. She felt she had struggled long and hard, and if she passed

WEEK 8

up her offer, all her efforts would have been useless. In fact, she felt she had to do it all herself. Her husband took the new position, and Joan stayed behind and began her career. She felt alone and abandoned and sought solace in food. Although her decision to remain proved to be a plus for her career, it created enormous stress on the marriage. Her husband got involved in an affair that almost led to divorce.

EXERCISE 1

1. Do you think your weight problems were caused by stress in your marriage?

_____

If the answer is yes, describe how.

_____

_____

2. Do you think your weight problems caused stress in your marriage?

_____

If the answer is yes, describe how.

_____

_____

3. How has your spouse influenced your weight gain?

_____

4. What does your spouse do now that makes your weight management efforts more difficult?

_____

EXERCISE 2

1. List changes you feel will make your marriage healthier and stronger.

_____

_____

_____

_____

_____

2. Have you discussed these possible changes with your spouse?

_____

3. What was the response?

_____

4. When will you initiate these changes?

_____

5. How will you make these changes?

_____

Over the next few months, notice if you are able to resolve issues in your relationship with your spouse more directly rather than resorting to food.

EXERCISE 3

1. What life-changing decisions have you made without prayerfully seeking God's will?

_____

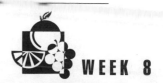

WEEK 8

2. What effects did such decisions have on your life? The lives of others close to you?

_____

_____

3. Do you still try to do it all yourself rather than seeking the Lord's will through prayer?

_____

_____

4. What are your feelings now as you imagine yourself following more closely to God's will and not just your own (e.g., peace, confidence, anxiety, apprehension)?

_____

_____

Stress Attacks Your Body on All Levels

According to findings reported in *Lancet,* the healing process may speed up if psychological stress eases. Researchers compared two groups of women who had undergone a punch biopsy, or small wound, in the forearm. One group faced severe daily stress; they were principal caregivers of dysfunctional relatives. The women, on average, required nine days longer to heal than the noncaregivers. The dramatic difference in healing time suggests that patients could benefit greatly from anxiety-reducing therapy before undergoing surgery.

Whether or not surgery is in your future, the importance of increasing your body's healing power is clear. Review the *Gentle Eating Workbook,* and implement as many of the stress reducers as you can into your daily activities. A good way to begin would be to listen to the *Gentle Eating* audiotape, or view the *Gentle Eating* videotape.

Remember to update and rearrange your activities from time to time to reduce stress and avoid boredom. Focus on pursuing wholesome activities that turn your thoughts from food.

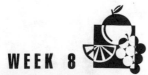

WEEK 8

PHYSICAL:
Reminder: Begin Exercise Routines Early to Kick-Start Metabolism!

Performing a variety of moderate physical activities can prevent exercise boredom. Listed are some gentle exercises to keep you moving through your day:

Morning
- Light stretching and bending—two minutes
- Exercise bike or walking—five minutes
- Extra stairs or steps—three minutes

Noon
- Walking or exercise bike—ten minutes

Evening
- Lifting light weights—five minutes
- Walking or swimming—ten minutes
- Exercise bike or light stretching and bending—five minutes

Household Chores Can "Sweep" Away Calories

If you itemized some of your favorite activities, whether the list was short or long, chances are that "doing household chores" would not make the cut. However, a report appearing in the *Orange County Register* (October 18, 1995) provides some interesting statistics:

Over time, given constant but moderate physical activity, you can develop a stronger, leaner body, boost your energy, relieve your stress and burn hundreds of calories an hour. And you can get that physical activity right at home, doing household chores. For example, a 180-pound man burns 522 calories an hour scrubbing floors and tubs;

WEEK 8

for a 130-pound woman, it's 377. A 180-pound man in an hour can burn 306 calories mopping, 288 calories washing windows, 234 calories sweeping. A 130-pound woman in an hour can burn 162 calories vacuuming, 144 calories dusting and 114 calories ironing. It's not just the calorie-burning that makes these activities worthwhile; it's the stretching and strengthening. It's the focus you bring to the activity, the conscious awareness of moving fully and breathing deeply that, over time, can add to your fitness.

Okay. Perhaps the information is not enough to entice you into doing windows, but keep it in mind!

Train Your Children; Stop the Food Problem Chain

Encourage children to pay attention to their natural hunger signals. Usually, children will tell you how much, if any, food they want. If they say they are not hungry, do not force them to eat, and never make children eat food they do not like.

Whenever practical, allow children to choose food they want and the portion size. Then teach them to eat slowly until they are no longer hungry (not full). Show them by example how to wait a few minutes to let food reach their stomachs and signal their brains whether they are still hungry. Once they determine they are no longer hungry, any food not eaten should be left on their plates. Leftovers can be refrigerated, but as you become more aware of your children's food preferences, leftovers should not be a problem. If a main dish is not preferred, allow your children to choose a healthy alternative from categories you determine, such as cereal, fruit, or yogurt.

The goal is to prevent an obsession with eating. Keep food a non-emotional issue and your children will learn early to eat to have fuel, not to cope.

This week try to

- teach your children to rate their hunger (0 = starved; 5 = satisfied; 10 = stuffed) by listening to their hunger signals.

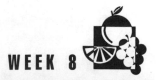

- have your children estimate how much food they need not to be hungry.
- begin with an average portion of food: one-half cup or one cup.
- write down your thoughts and feelings about seeing food remaining on the plates.

What disposition did you make of the remaining food? Overall, it is less stressful to toss leftovers than to overeat and abuse yourself.

EXERCISE 1

1. I eat seconds because (check all that apply)

   __ I am hungry.
   __ food tastes good.
   __ it is a habit.
   __ I can't stand to waste food.
   __ food is available, so I eat.
   __ I feel I should not keep eating, so I rebel.
   __ Other: _____.

2. Feelings and thoughts I have as I anticipate not taking seconds are

   _____.

3. Consequences of eating as much as I need not to be hungry are

   _____.

4. At this point, I believe I cannot eat seconds

   __   20 percent of the time because _____.
   __   40 percent of the time because _____.
   __   60 percent of the time because _____.
   __   90 percent of the time because _____.
   __   100 percent of the time because _____.

WEEK 8

EXERCISE 2

Think back over the past eight weeks, and recall all the tips you can remember to curb overeating

At home: _____

_____

While shopping: _____

_____

At family get-togethers: _____

_____

At social gatherings: _____

_____

While restaurant dining: _____

_____

At fast-food places: _____

_____

While traveling: _____

_____

At work: _____

_____

PROGRESS CHART

Check all that apply.

Spiritual Changes

___ Had at least a fifteen-minute daily quiet time.

___ Memorized a Bible verse.

___ Met with midweek church group.

___ Went to church services.

___ Prayed.

___ Felt a little closer to the Lord.

___ Expressed true feelings to God.

___ Honestly evaluated my relationship with God.

Thinking Changes

___ Recognized and recorded a distorted thought.

___ Experienced change in how I view myself.

___ Experienced change in how I thought about a situation.

___ Was able to develop more accurate/balanced view of person, event, etc.

Emotional Changes

___ Recorded my feelings.

___ Evaluated feelings before eating.

___ Expressed feelings in appropriate manner.

___ Noticed impact a person, place, or event had on my urge to eat.

___ Identified a past trauma or hurt.

___ Sought support from a trusted person.

___ Expressed hurt or pain in appropriate way.

___ Noticed how past hurt was related to urge to eat.

___ Worked on a stage of grief.

___ Noticed a change in level of a negative emotion.

___ Noticed a different reaction to person, place, or event that used to evoke emotional upset.

___ Implemented clear, personal emotional boundaries.

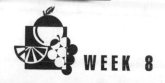

WEEK 8

PROGRESS CHART

Check all that apply.

Physical/Behavioral Changes

___ Charted my eating patterns.

___ Did workbook exercises.

___ Tried a new low-fat recipe.

___ Performed at least ten minutes of physical activity.

___ Listened to or watched ten to twenty minutes of a relaxation tape (audio or video).

___ Took at least fifteen minutes for myself.

___ Left some food on my plate.

___ Set a nice table with special touches: flowers, tablecloth, candles; listened to soothing music during mealtime; used special dishes.

___ Went shopping when not hungry.

___ Ate intended portions and stopped.

___ Rated hunger level before and after meals.

WEEK 8

CONCLUSION

by Dr. Vivian Lamphear

■ We are sure you have emerged happier and healthier from your journey through this workbook. No doubt you have accomplished significant changes during the past eight weeks. Congratulations on your progress!

Since this workbook was designed to be a continuing reference, you might want to review your thoughts and answers to the exercises and update them from time to time. It should prove interesting to note personal growth and positive results in all areas as you adopt the STEP plan as a life plan.

Many of our Gentle Eating group members reported that changes made in their spiritual walk, thinking, emotions, and physical habits enabled them to gain insight into their food-related problems. The gentle, holistic STEP approach provided motivation for staying with their weight management program. Some felt that belonging to a support group helped them stay accountable and provided a place to practice their skills; however, it is not necessary to join a support group to reap benefits from the STEP plan.

Perhaps part of your journey produced pain from a source you had not identified or thought was better left hidden. However, by understanding the source of your pain and facing it, you may now be able to excise it from your life permanently.

For all of you who felt the need to experience a healthier, more rewarding lifestyle, we trust this workbook has aided you, and our prayer is that you continue to harvest a lifetime of healthy benefits—STEP by STEP.

Above all, stay close to God, and be gentle with yourself and others.

A P P E N D I X   A

Starting a
Gentle Eating Group

1. Start each meeting with a prayer. Then review guidelines for the group to remind the regular attendees and instruct the new ones.

   A. Avoid cross-talk, or counseling one another, unless it's part of the particular exercise.

   B. Avoid advising or correcting one another.

   C. To make sure everyone has an opportunity, let the group know they will have three to five minutes of share time. If their sharing becomes too lengthy, agree beforehand on a time-out signal to help them close their share time.

   D. Avoid talking about specific foods that may lead to bingeing after the meeting or during the week.

   E. Avoid any comments that would be shaming to the group or specific members since many overeaters are struggling with shame.

   F. Make members aware of the time frame for the group. To be effective, the group should meet for no longer than one and a half hours and for no less than one hour. If the meeting exceeds the scheduled time, participants may enjoy the evening but may not show up the next week because they felt they were out too late or for too long previously. These boundaries are important because many overeaters fail to set boundaries.

G. Get the name of each group attendee and follow up with a telephone call during the week. This helps build an excellent repeat attendance, which makes for a good group. Otherwise, you well may experience a "revolving door" without seeing results, which is very discouraging.

2. Tips.

A. Read the material in the *Gentle Eating Workbook* and plan each week carefully. Without dominating your group members, show them you are knowledgeable and are prepared to be a responsible leader.

B. Set low-pressure goals and put in place an accountability system. Again, structure will be key!

C. Encourage members to trade telephone numbers and call each other for support during difficult times. Avoid developing too many close relationships too soon, which might put members at risk for a relapse. Remember, you are learning boundaries and what are safe and unsafe territories.

D. Be sensitive, but don't counsel those that may need professional therapy in addition to the group. Let members know it is okay to seek appropriate counseling. For a free evaluation or referral, call 1-800-NEW-LIFE. You will notice that people with bulimia, anorexia nervosa, and daily binge eating frequent these types of groups. Don't counsel them yourself. Set your own boundaries and encourage group members to call for help in general if they feel the need.

3. Fun Things to Do.

A. Once in a while, plan a potluck dinner and ask everyone to bring a Gentle Eating dish. You will be teaching them how to entertain and have fun without relapsing.

B. Ask everyone to meet for lunch or dinner at a "safe" cafe and enjoy a low-fat meal. Afterward, take a trip to the mall and suggest that everyone buy a small gift to celebrate the healthy efforts.

C. Organize partners for group walks or runs based on each person's exercise level. Learn how to play together.

D. Trade new conversion recipes with each other and start a group recipe book using index cards. Be creative.

E. Recognize members who are experiencing weight loss with small gifts or rewards without shaming another member.

F. Constantly remind your group of this truth: they are not being deprived, but are living and eating better with the Gentle Eating plan.

G. Always close in prayer asking for God's grace, power, and His will to be done in each person's life. Grace with accountability is important.

APPENDIX B

Guidelines for a Gentle Eating Group

■ A Gentle Eating group is a self-help group with an appointed group leader. It will do no more for a person than the person is willing to do individually. For the group to work well, there needs to be a healthy balance of frank speaking and encouragement. This weekly meeting should provide a safe place where we come together to share our victories and disappointments, hurts and struggles. The following guidelines are designed to help start and facilitate a Gentle Eating group.

1. We should come together realizing that each weight problem is unique, whether brought on by overeating, heredity, or environment. We may not have caused ourselves to be overweight, but we must accept responsibility to be the best we can be with what we have.

2. Each person in the Gentle Eating group must be encouraged to accept responsibility to change and to make responsible decisions. We are sometimes cut off from vital relationships because of our past actions, which may have been irresponsible. The group is an invitation to change that.

3. By our nature we may shrug off or attempt to cover up our problems; however, our weight is actually one way we are showing our pain. James 5:16 says for us to confess our sins to each other to

experience healing. This group should become a safe place where we can open up and share who we are and what we are experiencing. This is the place to make the journey from secrecy to openness. Let the light of openness and understanding flood the dark corners of our minds. Secrets die when brought to light.

The group should encourage openness to others outside the group.

4. The group should always last one to one and one-half hours, beginning and ending on time.

Time should be taken to go around the room and allow participants to state how much they weigh, how much they lost or gained that week, and their goal for the next week. Participants should be encouraged to weigh only once a week and, also, keep track of inches lost around the waist, thighs, and chest. If participants do not want to share this information initially, they should be given that choice. The hope is that they will see the value of being open.

(A facilitator should bring a good scale to the group each week. Anyone showing consistent weight loss should be recognized by the group. Encourage someone who lost too much in too little time to proceed more slowly. In all that we do, we should reinforce gradual changes and gentle treatment of self and others.)

5. While the group will be a safe place for us each week to share our feelings, emphasis should always be placed on what we are going to do about those feelings. Action is the focus. Encourage each person to do something positive and responsible each week.

6. Often we hear about food in a group and it causes us to obsess over that food. Try to eliminate as much talk about food as possible. Focus on feelings and actions. If food is discussed, be sure it is a nonfat food that someone has discovered and has rated high in taste and appetite satisfaction.

7. While the group is in session, it is important that side conversations do not occur. This prevents us from being distracted. The facilita-

tor may have to take a firm stand with those who insist on having private conversations during the meeting.

8. Above all, confidentiality must be maintained. What is said there, stays there. Ask each person who joins to commit to keeping all information and names of attendees strictly confidential.

9. Each person who comes to the group needs to commit to eight weeks of attendance. Many excuses to quit the group may crop up along the way. Making a commitment will help us stay involved even during the rough spots.

10. Be sure that each group meeting ends with everyone holding hands and saying the Lord's Prayer, the Serenity Prayer, or someone leading a personal prayer.

BIBLIOGRAPHY

Beck, Aaron T., and Gary Emery with Ruth L. Greenberg. *Anxiety Disorders and Phobias: A Cognitive Perspective*. New York: Basic, 1985.

Beck, Aaron T., A. John Rush, Brian F. Shaw, and Gary Emery. *Cognitive Therapy of Depression*. New York: Guilford, 1979.

Billigmeier, Shirley. *Inner Eating*. Nashville: Thomas Nelson, 1991.

Bradshaw, John. *Homecoming*. New York: Bantam, 1990.

Burns, David D. *The Feeling Good Handbook*. New York: Morrow, 1989.

Connor, Sonja L., and William E. Connor. *The New American Diet*. New York: Simon & Schuster, 1986.

Hammond, D. Corydon, ed. *Handbook of Hypnotic Suggestions and Metaphors*. An American Society of Clinical Hypnosis Book 1. New York: Norton, 1990.

The Life Recovery Bible. The Living Bible. Wheaton: Tyndale, 1992.

Possibility Thinkers Bible. The New King James Version. Nashville: Thomas Nelson, 1984.

Whitfield, Charles L. *Boundaries and Relationships*. Deerfield Beach: Health Communications, 1993.

ABOUT THE AUTHORS

Stephen Arterburn, M.Ed., is cofounder and chairman of the Minirth Meier New Life Clinics, which has more than one hundred clinics in operation across the nation. He is currently host of the Minirth Meier New Life Clinic radio program with a listening audience of more than one million. He is a nationally known speaker and has been a regular guest on nationally syndicated television talk shows. He is the author or coauthor of eighteen books, including *Winning at Work Without Losing at Love, The Angry Man, Addicted to "Love,"* and *Faith That Hurts, Faith That Heals*. Arterburn holds degrees from Baylor University and the University of North Texas and has been awarded two honorary doctorate degrees. In 1993 he was named Socially Responsible Entrepreneur of the Year by *Inc. Magazine,* Ernst and Young, and Merrill Lynch. Arterburn and his wife, Sandy, and daughter, Madeline, live in Laguna Beach, California.

Dr. Vivian Lamphear is a clinical psychologist and the director of the Lamphear Counseling Center with offices in Los Alamitos and Newport Beach, California. She is a popular radio cohost, lecturer, and author. Dr. Lamphear is a former assistant professor and child clinic director specializing in permanent weight loss, trauma, anger control, and parenting. She lives in southern California with her husband, Ken, and their two children, Ryanna and Dylan.

Sherry Marlar is a freelance writer, editor, and speaker based in Huntington Beach, California.

BOOKS BY STEPHEN ARTERBURN

Addicted to "Love" (Servant)

The Angry Man, Arterburn and David Stoop (Word)

The Complete Life Encyclopedia, Arterburn, Frank Minirth, M.D., and Paul Meier, M.D. (Thomas Nelson)

Drug-Proof Your Kids, Arterburn and Jim Burns (Focus on the Family; re-released by Gospel Light)

Faith That Hurts, Faith That Heals (originally titled *Toxic Faith*) Arterburn and Jack Felton (Thomas Nelson)

52 Simple Ways to Say "I Love You," Arterburn and Carl Dreizler (Thomas Nelson)

Gentle Eating, Arterburn, Mary Ehemann, and Vivian Lamphear, Ph.D. (Thomas Nelson)

Growing Up Addicted (Ballantine)

Hand-Me-Down Genes and Second-Hand Emotions (hardcover: Thomas Nelson; paperback as *Hand Me Down Genes:* Simon & Schuster)

How Will I Tell My Mother?, Arterburn and Jerry Arterburn (Thomas Nelson)

The Life Recovery Bible, Arterburn and David Stoop, executive editors (Tyndale)

Miracle Drugs, Arterburn, Frank Minirth, M.D., and Paul Meier, M.D. (Thomas Nelson)

The Power Book, Arterburn (Thomas Nelson)

The 12 Step Life Recovery Devotional, Arterburn and David Stoop (Tyndale)

When Love Is Not Enough, Arterburn and Jim Burns (hardcover and paperback as *Steering Them Straight:* Focus on the Family)

When Someone You Love Is Someone You Hate, Arterburn and David Stoop (Word)

Winning at Work Without Losing at Love (Thomas Nelson)

If you can't find one of these books in your local bookstore, you may order it through 1-800-BOOKS45.

To purchase the Finding the Power to Win audio and video series, phone 1-800-528-3825.